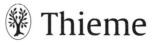

Pocket Atlas of Sectional Anatomy

Computed Tomography and Magnetic Resonance Imaging

Volume I
Head and Neck

Torsten B. Moeller, MD
Department of Radiology
Marienhaus Klinikum Saarlouis–Dillingen
Dillingen/Saarlouis, Germany

Emil Reif, MD
Department of Radiology
Marienhaus Klinikum Saarlouis–Dillingen
Dillingen/Saarlouis, Germany

4th edition

501 illustrations

Thieme
Stuttgart · New York

IV

Library of Congress Cataloging-in-Publication Data

Möller, Torsten B., author.

[Taschenatlas der Schnittbildanatomie. English]

Pocket atlas of sectional anatomy : computed tomography and magnetic resonance imaging / Torsten B. Moeller, Emil Reif. — Fourth edition.

p. ; cm.

This book is an authorized translation of the 3rd German edition published in 2011 by Georg Thieme Verlag, Stuttgart.

Includes bibliographical references and index.

ISBN 978-3-13-125504-4 (v. 1 : paperback : alk. paper) — ISBN 978-3-13-170844-1 (v. 1 : eISBN) -- ISBN 978-3-13-125604-1 (v. 2 : paperback : alk. paper) — ISBN 978-3-13-170854-0 (v. 2 : eISBN) — ISBN 978-3-13-143171-4 (v. 3 : paperback : alk. paper)

I. Reif, Emil, author. II. Title.

[DNLM: 1. Anatomy, Regional—Atlases. 2. Magnetic Resonance Imaging—Atlases. 3. Tomography, X-Ray Computed—Atlases. QS 17]

QM25

612.0022'2—dc23

2013029515

Original translation by Barbara Herzberger, MD, Munich, Germany. New parts translated by Terry C. Telger, Fort Worth, TX, USA

Illustrators: Torsten B. Moeller, Dillingen/Saarlouis, Germany; Barbara Gay, Stuttgart, Germany

3rd English edition 2006
3rd French edition 2008
3rd German edition 2005
2nd Greek edition 2002
3rd Japanese edition 2008
1st Korean edition 2010
2nd Portuguese-Brasilian edition 2009
3rd Spanish edition 2007
1st Turkish edition 2007

© 2014 Georg Thieme Verlag KG, Rüdigerstrasse 14, 70469 Stuttgart, Germany
http://www.thieme.de
Thieme Medical Publishers, Inc., 333 Seventh Avenue, New York, NY 10001, USA
http://www.thieme.com

Cover design: Thieme Publishing Group
Typesetting by primustype Robert Hurler GmbH, Notzingen, Germany
Printed in Germany by AZ Druck und Datentechnik GmbH
ISBN 978-3-13-125504-4

Also available as an e-book:
eISBN 978-3-13-170844-1

Important note: Medicine is an ever-changing science undergoing continual development. Research and clinical experience are continually expanding our knowledge, in particular our knowledge of proper treatment and drug therapy. Insofar as this book mentions any dosage or application, readers may rest assured that the authors, editors, and publishers have made every effort to ensure that such references are in accordance with **the state of knowledge at the time of production of the book.**

Nevertheless, this does not involve, imply, or express any guarantee or responsibility on the part of the publishers in respect to any dosage instructions and forms of applications stated in the book. **Every user is requested to examine carefully** the manufacturers' leaflets accompanying each drug and to check, if necessary in consultation with a physician or specialist, whether the dosage schedules mentioned therein or the contraindications stated by the manufacturers differ from the statements made in the present book. Such examination is particularly important with drugs that are either rarely used or have been newly released on the market. Every dosage schedule or every form of application used is entirely at the user's own risk and responsibility. The authors and publishers request every user to report to the publishers any discrepancies or inaccuracies noticed. If errors in this work are found after publication, errata will be posted at www.thieme.com on the product description page.

To Bernie and Arlene Riegner,
the roots of the American part
of my family, with love

Preface

The popularity of the *Pocket Atlas of Sectional Anatomy*, the many foreign-language translations that ensued, and the many positive responses and constructive criticisms were very gratifying for us and prompted us to make even more improvements to Volume I. Recent technical advances in magnetic resonance imaging have brought significant quality improvements, which are reflected in this volume. Many of the older images have been replaced, and many of the new images were produced with 3-Tesla scanners. We are grateful to the manufacturers, Siemens and Philips, for providing this technology.

The better spatial resolution has naturally allowed for a higher level of detail in the labeling of anatomic features. But at the same time, we wanted to preserve the character of the previous editions by keeping the book highly informative yet compact and easy to use. For some images, therefore, we decided to place a "magnified" view with additional labels on the facing page. We received a great deal of input on naming the spaces in the neck, and we did this separately, as we did for the vascular territories in the neurocranium.

We express special thanks to our radiology technologists and our fellow physicians, especially Eberhard Bauer, for providing us with excellent MDCT images.

Torsten B. Moeller
Emil Reif

Table of Contents

◼ Cranial CT

◼ Cranial MRI

◼ Neck

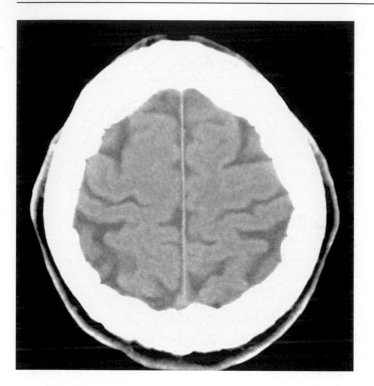

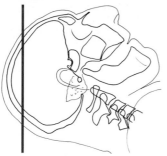

 Frontal lobe

Parietal lobe

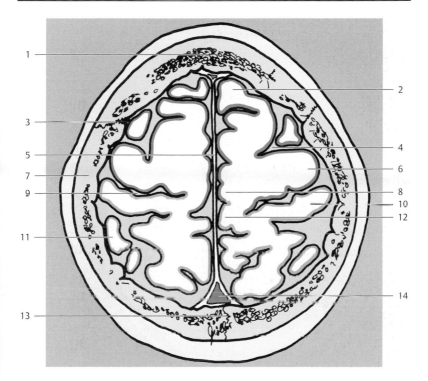

1 Frontal bone
2 Superior frontal gyrus
3 Coronal suture
4 Precentral sulcus
5 Falx cerebri
6 Precentral gyrus
7 Parietal bone
8 Paracentral lobule
9 Central sulcus
10 Postcentral gyrus
11 Superior parietal lobule
12 Precuneus
13 Sagittal suture
14 Superior sagittal sinus

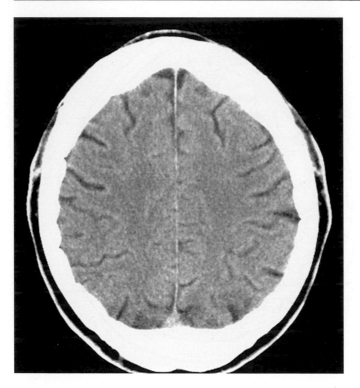

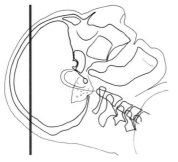

Frontal lobe
Parietal lobe

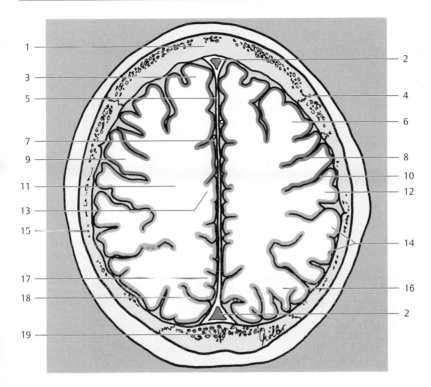

1 Frontal bone
2 Superior sagittal sinus
3 Superior frontal gyrus
4 Coronal suture
5 Falx cerebri
6 Middle frontal gyrus
7 Longitudinal cerebral fissure
8 Precentral sulcus
9 Precentral gyrus
10 Central sulcus
11 Cerebral white matter
    (semioval center)
12 Postcentral gyrus
13 Paracentral lobule
14 Supramarginal gyrus
15 Parietal bone
16 Inferior parietal lobule
17 Precuneus
18 Parieto-occipital sulcus
19 Occipital bone

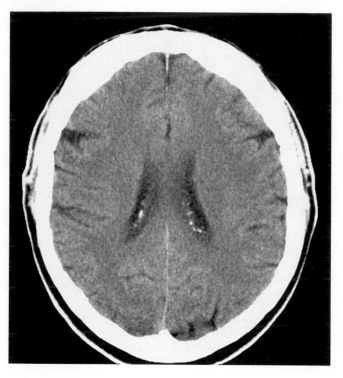

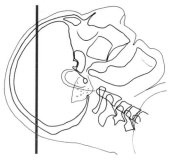

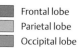

Frontal lobe
Parietal lobe
Occipital lobe

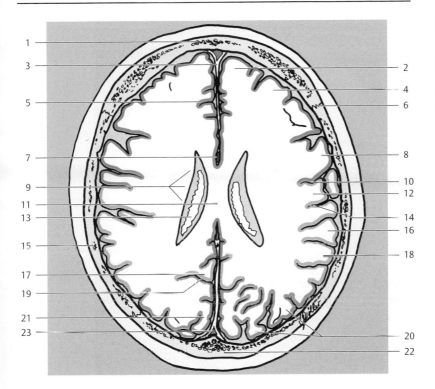

1 Frontal bone
2 Superior frontal gyrus
3 Falx cerebri
4 Middle frontal gyrus
5 Cingulate sulcus
6 Coronal suture
7 Pericallosal artery
8 Precentral gyrus
9 Corona radiata
10 Central sulcus
11 Corpus callosum
12 Postcentral gyrus
13 Lateral ventricle (choroid plexus)
14 Postcentral sulcus
15 Parietal bone
16 Supramarginal gyrus
17 Precuneus
18 Angular gyrus
19 Parieto-occipital sulcus
20 Occipital gyri
21 Cuneus
22 Occipital bone
23 Superior sagittal sinus

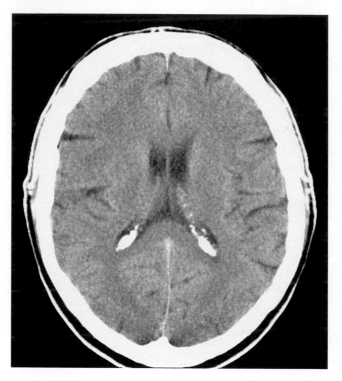

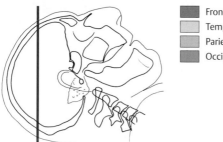

Frontal lobe
Temporal lobe
Parietal lobe
Occipital lobe

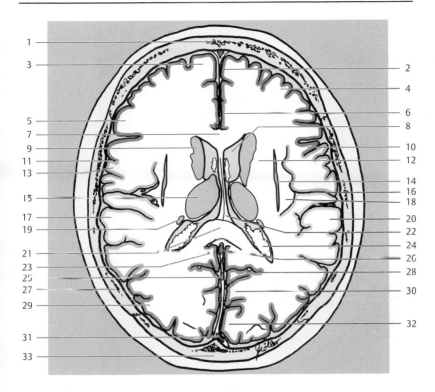

1   Frontal bone
2   Falx cerebri
3   Superior frontal gyrus
4   Middle frontal gyrus
5   Inferior frontal gyrus
6   Cingulate gyrus
7   Corpus callosum (trunk)
8   Lateral ventricle (anterior horn)
9   Caudate nucleus (head)
10 Precentral gyrus
11 Central sulcus
12 Corona radiata
13 Postcentral gyrus
14 Claustrum
15 Thalamus
16 Lateral sulcus
17 Temporal operculum
18 Insula
19 Caudate nucleus (tail)
20 Superior temporal gyrus
21 Corpus callosum (splenium)
22 Fornix
23 Cingulum
24 Lateral ventricle (collateral trigone, choroid plexus)
25 Straight sinus
26 Great cerebral vein (vein of Galen)
27 Parietal bone
28 Parieto-occipital sulcus
29 Occipital gyri
30 Cuneus
31 Superior sagittal sinus
32 Striate cortex
33 Occipital bone

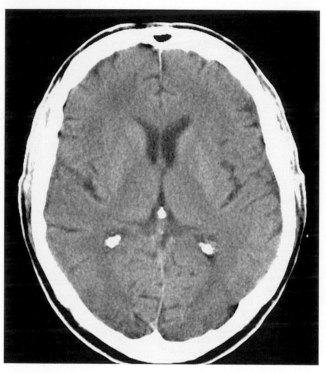

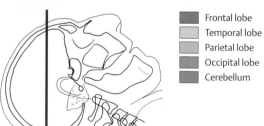

- ■ Frontal lobe
- □ Temporal lobe
- ▨ Parietal lobe
- ■ Occipital lobe
- ■ Cerebellum

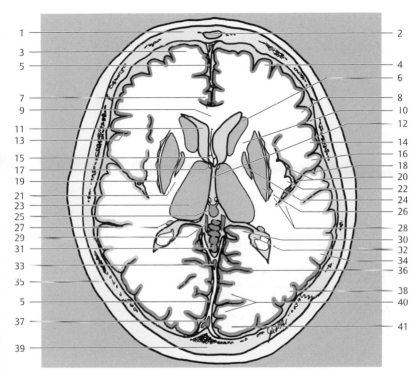

1 Frontal bone
2 Frontal sinus
3 Superior frontal gyrus
4 Middle frontal gyrus
5 Falx cerebri
6 Caudate nucleus (head)
7 Cingulate gyrus
8 Inferior frontal gyrus
9 Corpus callosum (genu)
10 Internal capsule (anterior limb)
11 Lateral ventricle (anterior horn)
12 Third ventricle
13 Central sulcus
14 Precentral gyrus
15 Fornix
16 Postcentral gyrus
17 Interventricular foramen
   (foramen of Monro)
18 Lateral sulcus
19 Claustrum
20 Insular arteries in the cistern of
   lateral cerebral fossa (insular
   cistern)

21 Internal capsule (posterior limb)
22 Insula
23 Thalamus
24 Globus pallidus (pallidum)
25 Pineal gland
26 Putamen
27 Caudate nucleus (tail)
28 Transverse temporal gyrus
29 Internal cerebral vein
30 Hippocampus
31 Vermis of cerebellum
32 Lateral ventricle (trigone with
   choroid plexus)
33 Straight sinus
34 Middle temporal gyrus
35 Parietal bone
36 Parieto-occipital sulcus
37 Superior sagittal sinus
38 Occipital gyri
39 Occipital bone
40 Striate cortex
41 Occipital pole

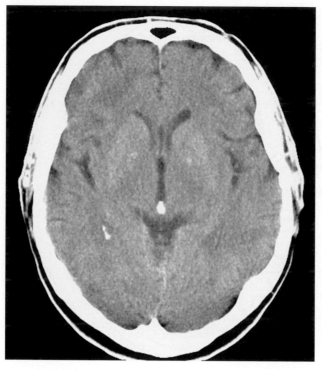

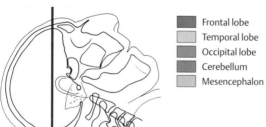

■ Frontal lobe
☐ Temporal lobe
■ Occipital lobe
■ Cerebellum
☐ Mesencephalon

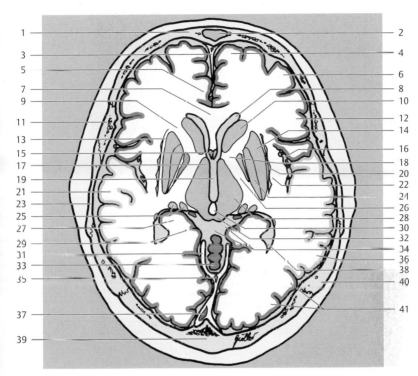

1 Frontal bone
2 Frontal sinus
3 Falx cerebri
4 Superior frontal gyrus
5 Cingulate gyrus
6 Middle frontal gyrus
7 Corpus callosum (genu)
8 Lateral ventricle (anterior horn)
9 Internal capsule (anterior limb)
10 Caudate nucleus (head)
11 Parietal bone
12 Inferior frontal gyrus
13 External capsule
14 Putamen
15 Septum verum
   (precommissural septum)
16 Cistern of lateral cerebral fossa
   (insular cistern)
17 Hypothalamus
18 Internal capsule (genu)
19 Third ventricle
20 Claustrum
21 Superior temporal gyrus
22 Extreme capsule
23 Temporal bone
24 Globus pallidus (pallidum)
25 Geniculate body
26 Internal capsule (posterior limb)
27 Hippocampus
28 Thalamus
29 Parahippocampal gyrus
30 Pineal gland (calcified)
31 Tentorium cerebelli
32 Quadrigeminal plate (colliculus)
33 Vermis of cerebellum
34 Quadrigeminal and ambient cisterns
35 Straight sinus
36 Middle temporal gyrus
37 Superior sagittal sinus
38 Lateral ventricle (trigone)
39 Occipital bone
40 Parietal bone
41 Occipital gyri

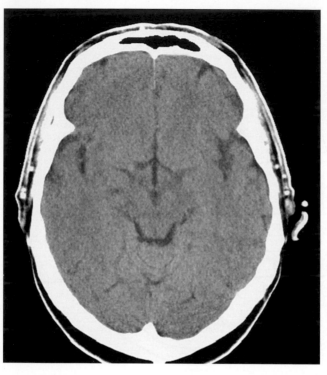

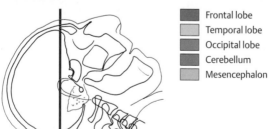

Frontal lobe
Temporal lobe
Occipital lobe
Cerebellum
Mesencephalon

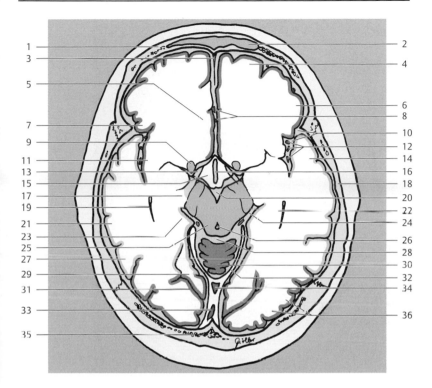

1 Frontal bone
2 Frontal sinus
3 Falx cerebri
4 Superior frontal gyrus
5 Cingulate gyrus
6 Middle frontal gyrus
7 Inferior frontal gyrus
8 Anterior cerebral artery
9 Striatum (inferior portion)
10 Lateral sulcus (insular cistern)
11 Insula
12 Insular arteries
13 Optic tract
14 Superior temporal gyrus
15 Hypothalamus
16 Third ventricle
17 Cerebral peduncle
18 Parietal bone
19 Lateral ventricle (temporal horn)
20 Interpeduncular cistern
21 Middle temporal gyrus
22 Hippocampus
23 Parahippocampal gyrus
24 Ambient cistern
25 Mesencephalon (quadrigeminal plate)
26 Aqueduct
27 Inferior temporal gyrus
28 Quadrigeminal cistern
29 Lateral occipitotemporal gyrus
30 Vermis of cerebellum (superior portion)
31 Parieto-occipital sulcus
32 Tentorium cerebelli
33 Superior sagittal sinus
34 Straight sinus
35 Occipital bone
36 Occipital gyri

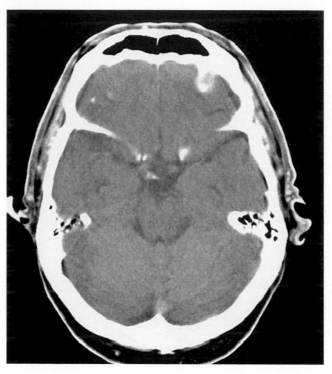

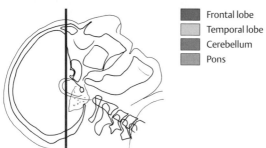

Frontal lobe
Temporal lobe
Cerebellum
Pons

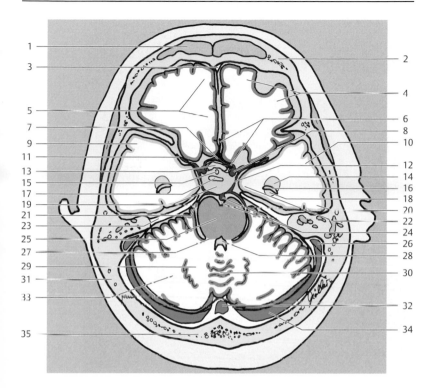

1 Frontal sinus
3 Falx cerebri
5 Straight gyrus
7 Anterior communicating artery
9 Superior temporal gyrus
11 Middle cerebral artery
13 Optic chiasm
15 Pituitary stalk
17 Dorsum sellae
19 Pentagon of basal cisterns
21 Posterior cerebral artery
23 Tentorium cerebelli
25 Pons
27 Cerebellar peduncle (middle)
29 Dentate nucleus
31 Temporal bone
33 Cerebellar hemisphere
35 Occipital bone

 1 Frontal sinus
 2 Frontal bone
 3 Falx cerebri
 4 Orbital gyri
 5 Straight gyrus
 6 Anterior cerebral artery
 7 Anterior communicating artery
 8 Internal carotid artery
 9 Superior temporal gyrus
10 Middle temporal gyrus
11 Middle cerebral artery
12 Posterior communicating
   artery
13 Optic chiasm
14 Amygdaloid body
15 Pituitary stalk
16 Lateral ventricle
   (temporal horn)
17 Dorsum sellae
18 Hippocampus
19 Pentagon of basal cisterns
20 Inferior temporal gyrus
21 Posterior cerebral artery
22 Parahippocampal gyrus
23 Tentorium cerebelli
24 Basilar artery and basal sulcus
25 Pons
26 Sigmoid sinus
27 Cerebellar peduncle (middle)
28 Fourth ventricle
29 Dentate nucleus
30 Vermis of cerebellum
   (superior part)
31 Temporal bone
32 Confluence of the sinuses
33 Cerebellar hemisphere
34 Transverse sinus
35 Occipital bone

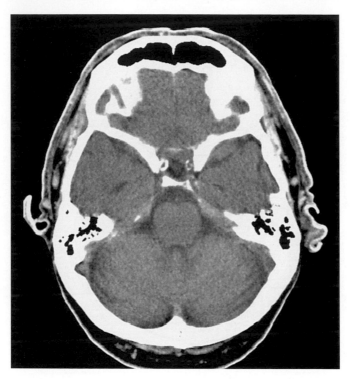

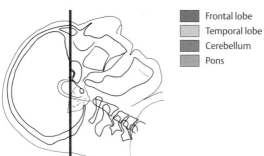

■ Frontal lobe
□ Temporal lobe
■ Cerebellum
■ Pons

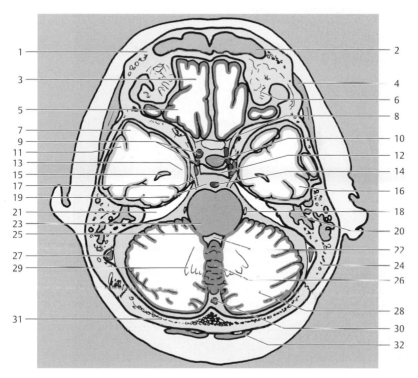

1 Frontal bone	17 Trigeminal nerve (V)
2 Frontal sinus	18 Trochlear nerve (IV)
3 Straight gyrus	19 Pontine cistern
4 Temporal muscle	20 Mastoid antrum
5 Orbital gyri	21 Tentorium cerebelli
6 Roof of orbit	22 Fourth ventricle
7 Superior temporal gyrus	23 Pons
8 Optic nerve (II)	24 Temporal bone
9 Internal carotid artery	25 Cerebellar peduncle
10 Pituitary gland	26 Vermis of cerebellum
11 Middle temporal gyrus	27 Sigmoid sinus
12 Dorsum sellae	28 Cerebellar hemisphere
13 Parahippocampal gyrus	29 Dentate nucleus
14 Basilar artery	30 Occipital sinus
15 Lateral ventricle (temporal horn)	31 Occipital bone
16 Inferior temporal gyrus	32 Semispinalis capitis muscle

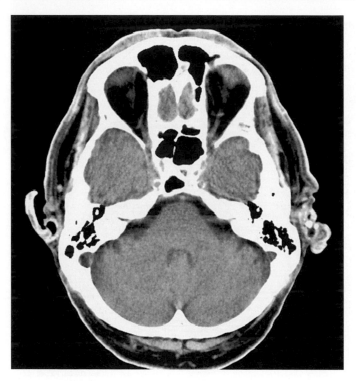

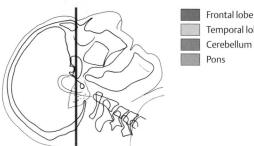

Frontal lobe
Temporal lobe
Cerebellum
Pons

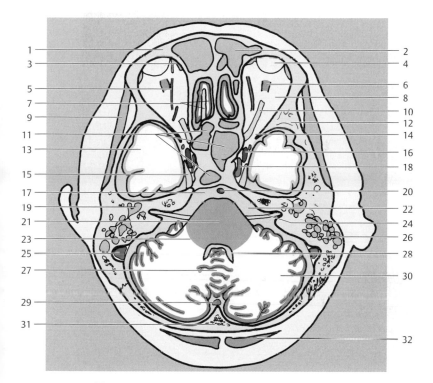

1 Frontal bone
2 Frontal sinus
3 Superior oblique muscle
4 Eyeball
5 Ophthalmic vein
6 Superior rectus muscle
7 Straight gyrus and olfactory bulb
8 Retro-orbital fatty tissue
9 Temporal muscle
10 Optic nerve (II)
11 Sphenoidal sinus
12 Sphenoidal bone
13 Inferior temporal gyrus
14 Superior orbital fissure
15 Trigeminal nerve (ganglion)
16 Internal carotid artery
17 Pontine cistern
18 Cavernous sinus
19 Mastoid antrum
20 Basilar artery
21 Pons
22 Pontocerebellar cistern
23 Middle and inferior cerebellar peduncle
24 Internal auditory meatus with facial (VII) and vestibulocochlear/acoustic (VIII) nerves
25 Sigmoid sinus
26 Mastoid process with mastoid cells
27 Vermis of cerebellum
28 Fourth ventricle
29 Occipital sinus
30 Cerebellar hemisphere
31 Occipital bone
32 Semispinalis capitis muscle

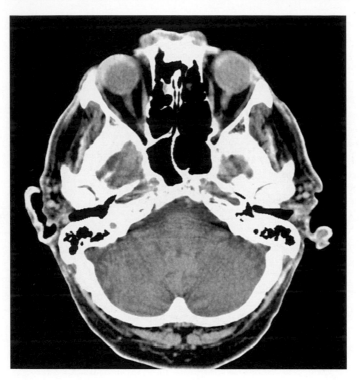

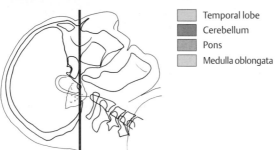

Temporal lobe
Cerebellum
Pons
Medulla oblongata

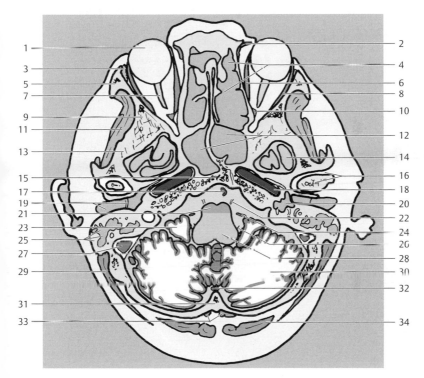

1 Eyeball
2 Superior oblique muscle
3 Lacrimal gland
4 Ethmoidal cells
5 Zygomatic bone
6 Medial rectus muscle
7 Optic nerve (II)
8 Lateral rectus muscle of eyeball
9 Sphenoidal bone
10 Superior rectus muscle
11 Temporal muscle
12 Sphenoidal sinus
13 Temporal bone
14 Temporal lobe (base)
15 Clivus
16 Temporomandibular joint and
    head of mandible
17 Basilar artery
18 Internal carotid artery
19 External auditory meatus and
    eardrum (tympanic membrane)
20 Tympanic cavity
21 Pons
22 Abducent nerve (VI)
23 Flocculus
24 Anterior inferior cerebellar artery
25 Mastoid process and mastoid cells
26 Glossopharyngeal (IX) and vagus (X)
    nerves
27 Sigmoid sinus
28 Medulla oblongata (myelencephalon)
29 Splenius capitis muscle
30 Cerebellar hemisphere
31 Occipital bone
32 Occipital sinus
33 Rectus capitis posterior minor muscle
34 Semispinalis capitis muscle

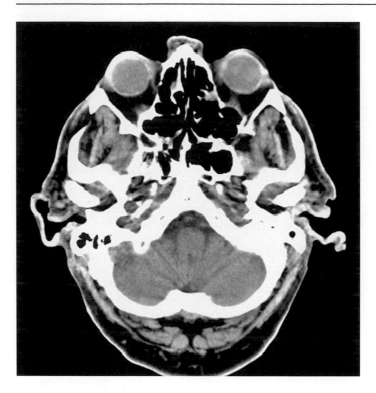

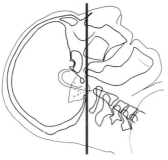

■ Cerebellum
☐ Medulla oblongata

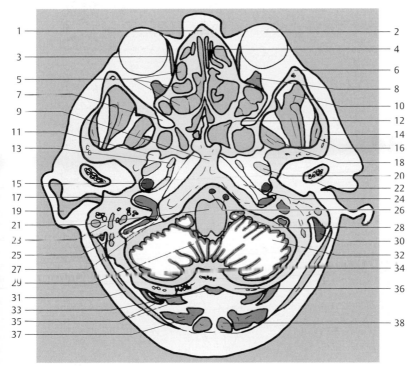

1	Nasal bone
2	Eyeball
3	Medial rectus muscle
4	Nasal septum
5	Ethmoidal cells
6	Zygomatic bone
7	Pterygopalatine fossa
8	Inferior rectus muscle
9	Occipital bone (basilar part)
10	Temporal muscle
11	Foramen ovale with mandibular nerve
12	Sphenoidal sinus
13	Temporal bone (apex of the petrous pyramid)
14	Zygomatic arch
15	Internal carotid artery
16	Masseter muscle
17	Jugular vein (bulb)
18	Lateral pterygoid muscle (superior head)
19	External auditory meatus
20	Auditory tube
21	Medulla oblongata
22	Head of mandible
23	Mastoid process
24	Foramen lacerum
25	Sigmoid sinus
26	Vertebral arteries
27	Petro-occipital fissure
28	Flocculus
29	Cerebellar tonsil
30	Digastric muscle
31	Splenius capitis muscle
32	Cerebellar hemisphere (caudal lobe)
33	Rectus capitis posterior minor muscle
34	Cisterna magna (posterior cerebello-medullary cistern)
35	Rectus capitis posterior major muscle
36	Occipital bone
37	Semispinalis capitis muscle
38	Trapezius muscle

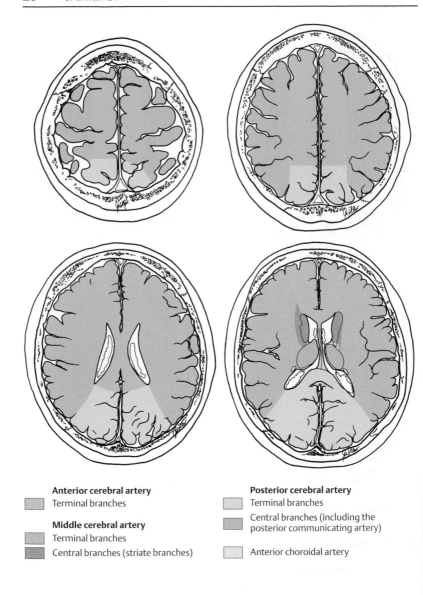

Anterior cerebral artery
Terminal branches

Middle cerebral artery
Terminal branches
Central branches (striate branches)

Posterior cerebral artery
Terminal branches
Central branches (including the posterior communicating artery)

Anterior choroidal artery

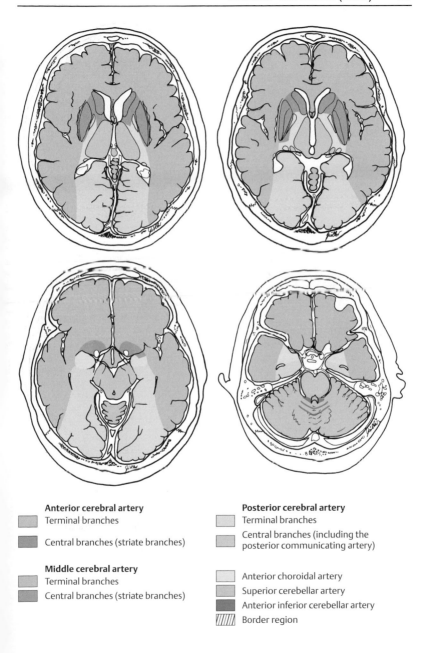

Anterior cerebral artery
Terminal branches

Central branches (striate branches)

Middle cerebral artery
Terminal branches

Central branches (striate branches)

Posterior cerebral artery
Terminal branches

Central branches (including the posterior communicating artery)

Anterior choroidal artery

Superior cerebellar artery

Anterior inferior cerebellar artery

Border region

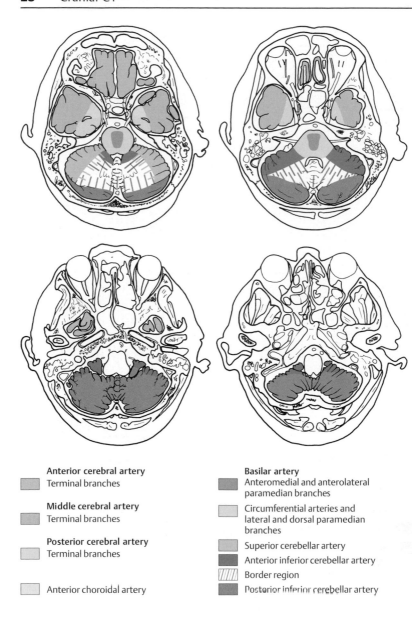

Anterior cerebral artery
Terminal branches

Middle cerebral artery
Terminal branches

Posterior cerebral artery
Terminal branches

Anterior choroidal artery

Basilar artery
Anteromedial and anterolateral paramedian branches

Circumferential arteries and lateral and dorsal paramedian branches

Superior cerebellar artery

Anterior inferior cerebellar artery

Border region

Posterior inferior cerebellar artery

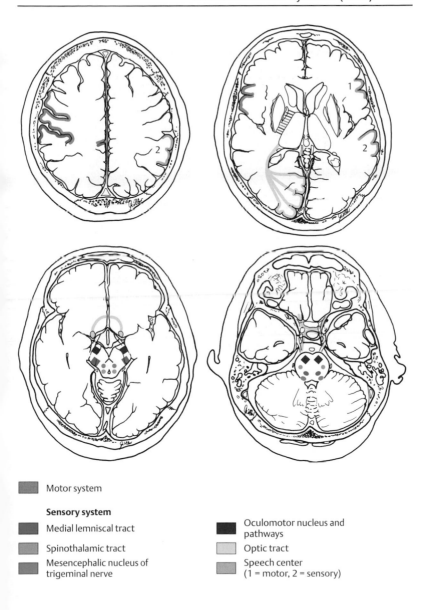

Motor system

Sensory system

Medial lemniscal tract

Spinothalamic tract

Mesencephalic nucleus of
trigeminal nerve

Oculomotor nucleus and
pathways

Optic tract

Speech center
(1 = motor, 2 = sensory)

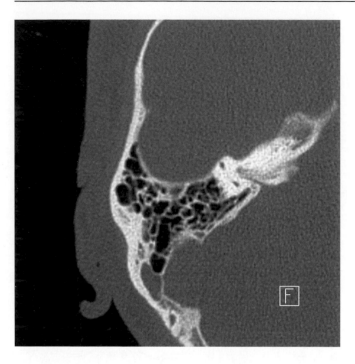

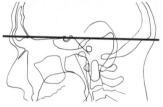

Frontal

Lateral ☐ Medial

Occipital

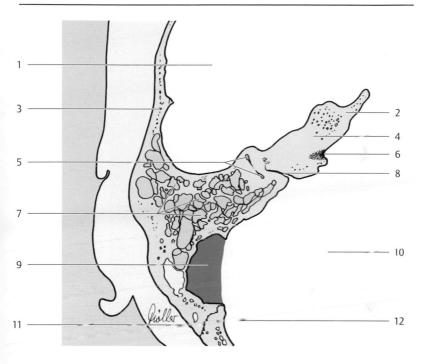

1 Middle cranial fossa
2 Petrous apex
3 Temporal bone, squamous part
4 Temporal bone, petrous part
5 Superior semicircular canal
6 Internal acoustic meatus
7 Mastoid cells
8 Vestibular aqueduct with endolymphatic duct
9 Sigmoid sinus
10 Posterior cranial fossa
11 Lambdoid suture
12 Occipital bone

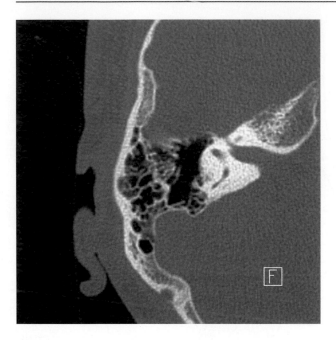

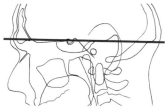

Frontal

Lateral ▢ Medial

Occipital

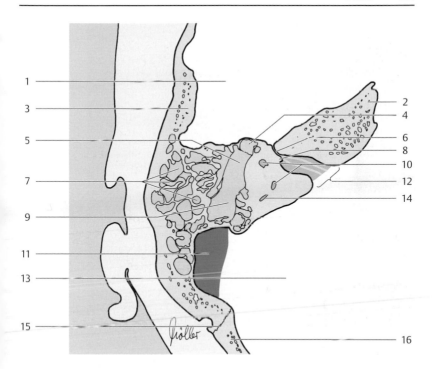

1 Middle cranial fossa
2 Petrous apex
3 Temporal bone, squamous part
4 Epitympanic recess (anterior)
5 Aditus ad antrum mastoideum
6 Facial nerve canal (VII)
7 Mastoid cells
8 Falciform crest
9 Mastoid antrum
10 Superior semicircular canal
11 Sigmoid sinus
12 Internal acoustic opening
13 Posterior cranial fossa
14 Posterior semicircular canal
15 Lambdoid suture
16 Occipital bone

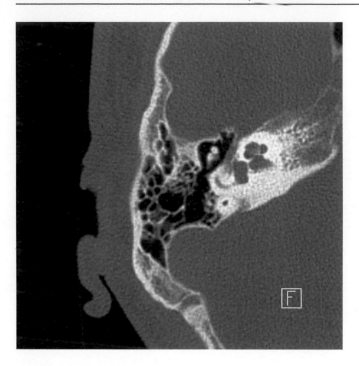

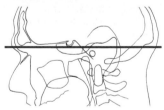

Frontal

Lateral ☐ Medial

Occipital

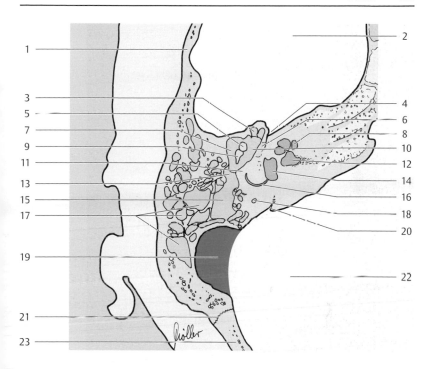

1 Temporal bone, squamous part
2 Middle cranial fossa
3 Epitympanic recess (anterior)
4 Hiatus for greater petrosal nerve
5 Malleus (head)
6 Facial nerve canal (VII), tympanic part
7 Epitympanic cavity (Prussak space)
8 Cochlea
9 Incus (lesser process)
10 Epitympanum
11 Promontory of basal turn of cochlea

12 Internal acoustic meatus
13 Aditus ad antrum mastoideum
14 Vestibule
15 Mastoid antrum
16 Lateral semicircular canal
17 Mastoid cells
18 Posterior semicircular canal
19 Sigmoid sinus
20 External opening of vestibular aqueduct
21 Lambdoid suture
22 Posterior cranial fossa
23 Occipital bone

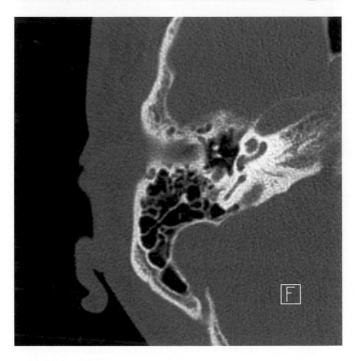

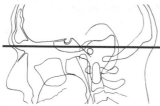

Frontal

Lateral ☐ Medial

Occipital

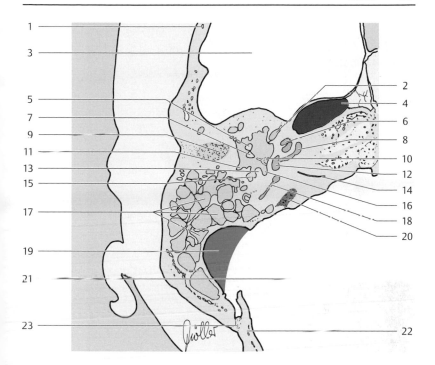

1 Temporal bone, squamous part
2 Tensor tympani muscle
3 Middle cranial fossa
4 Carotid canal
5 Malleus (manubrium)
6 Cochlea
7 Incus (body)
8 Basal turn of cochlea
9 External acoustic meatus
10 Stapes
11 Facial recess
12 Round window
13 Pyramidal eminence
14 Cochlear aqueduct
15 Facial nerve canal (VII, posterior genu)
16 Sinus tympani
17 Mastoid cells
18 Posterior semicircular canal
19 Sigmoid sinus
20 Jugular vein (bulb)
21 Posterior cranial fossa
22 Occipital bone
23 Lambdoid suture

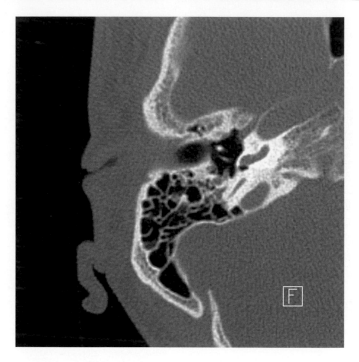

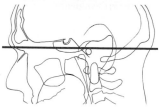

Frontal

Lateral ☐ Medial

Occipital

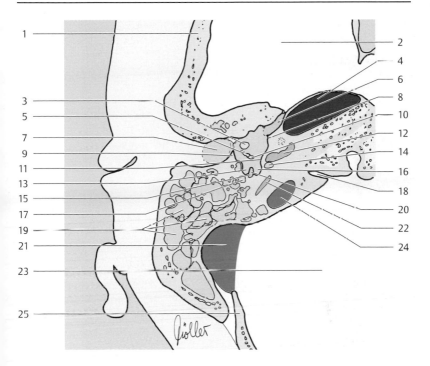

1 Temporal bone, squamous part
2 Middle cranial fossa
3 Malleus (manubrium)
4 Carotid canal
5 Incus (long crus and lenticular process)
6 Tensor tympani muscle
7 External acoustic meatus
8 Processus cochleariformis
9 Scutum
10 Stapes (head)
11 Promontory of basal turn of cochlea
12 Basal turn of cochlea
13 Facial nerve recess
14 Round window
15 Stapedius muscle
16 Sinus tympani
17 Facial nerve canal (VII), mastoid part
18 Cochlear aqueduct
19 Mastoid cells
20 Pyramidal eminence
21 Sigmoid sinus
22 Posterior semicircular canal
23 Posterior cranial fossa
24 Jugular vein (bulb)
25 Occipital bone

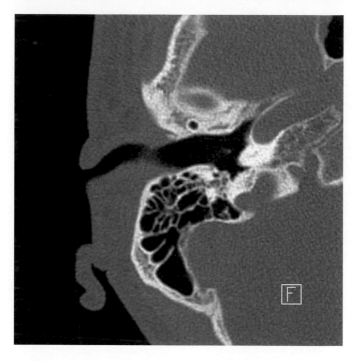

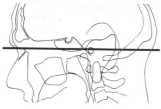

Frontal

Lateral ☐ Medial

Occipital

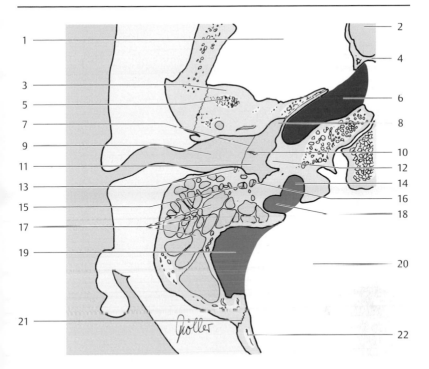

1 Middle cranial fossa
2 Sphenoidal sinus
3 Temporal bone, squamous part
4 Sphenoid
5 Temporomandibular joint (roof)
6 Carotid canal
7 Tympanic membrane
8 Auditory (eustachian) tube
9 External acoustic meatus
10 Malleus (manubrium)
11 Mesotympanum
12 Promontory (of basal turn of cochlea)
13 Tympanic nerve
14 Jugular foramen, pars nervosa
15 Facial nerve canal (VII), mastoid part
16 Stapedius
17 Mastoid cells
18 Jugular foramen, pars vascularis
19 Sigmoid sinus
20 Posterior cranial fossa
21 Lambdoid suture
22 Occipital bone

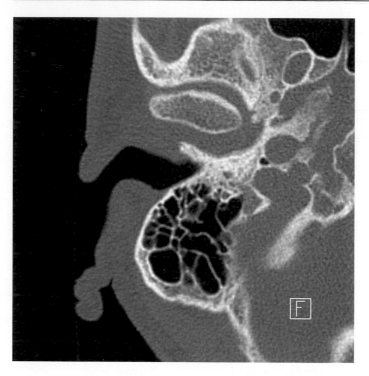

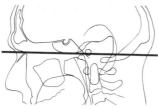

Frontal

Lateral ☐ Medial

Occipital

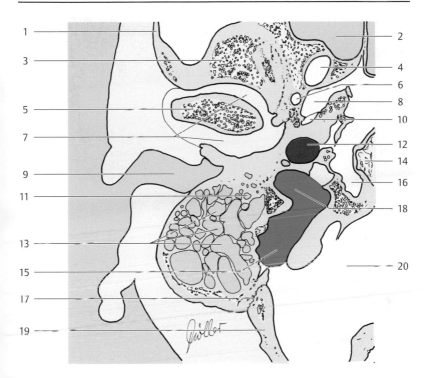

1 Zygomatic process
2 Sphenoidal sinus
3 Temporal bone with articular tubercle
4 Foramen ovale
5 Head of mandible
6 Foramen spinosum
7 Mandibular fossa
8 Foramen lacerum
9 External acoustic meatus
10 Pharyngotympanic tube (auditory tube)
11 Facial nerve canal (VII)
12 Internal carotid artery, petrous part (vertical segment)
13 Mastoid cells
14 Basiocciput (clivus, occipital bone)
15 Sigmoid sinus
16 Hypoglossal canal
17 Occipitomastoid suture
18 Jugular foramen
19 Occipital bone
20 Posterior cranial fossa

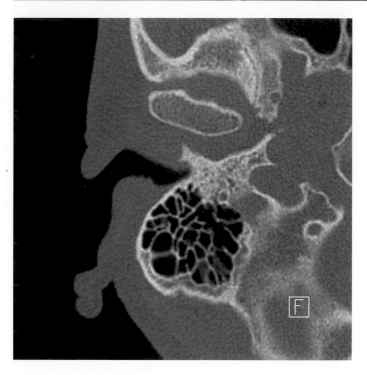

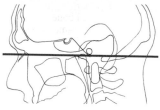

Frontal

Lateral ☐ Medial

Occipital

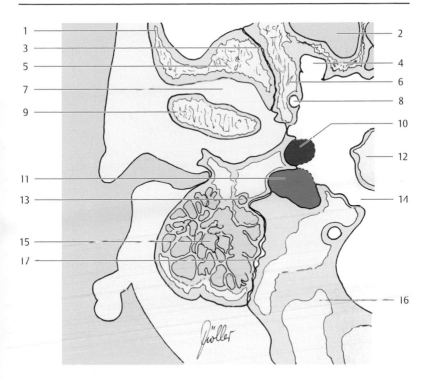

1 Zygomatic process
2 Sphenoidal sinus
3 Sphenosquamous suture
4 Foramen ovale
5 Temporal bone
6 Sphenoid
7 Temporomandibular joint
8 Foramen spinosum
9 Head of mandible
10 Internal carotid artery, petrous part (vertical segment)

11 Jugular foramen
12 Clivus, occipital bone
13 Stylomastoid foramen with facial nerve (VII)
14 Hypoglossal canal
15 Mastoid process
16 Occipital bone (occipital condyle)
17 Occipitomastoid suture

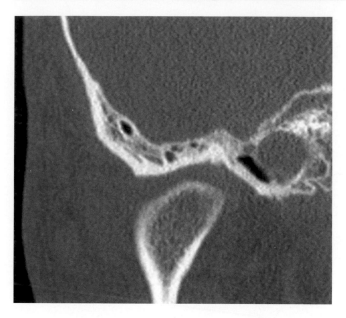

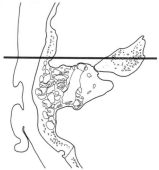

Cranial

Lateral ☐ Medial

Caudal

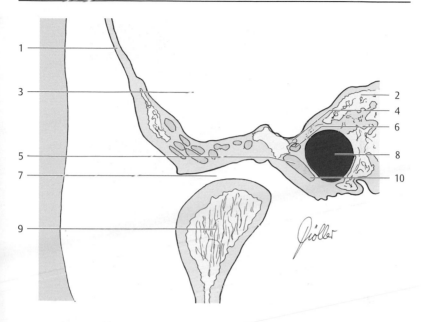

1 Temporal bone
2 Petrous apex
3 Middle cranial fossa
4 Geniculate ganglion
5 Mesotympanum
6 Tensor tympani muscle
7 Temporomandibular joint
8 Internal carotid artery, petrous part (horizontal segment)
9 Head of mandible
10 Hypotympanum

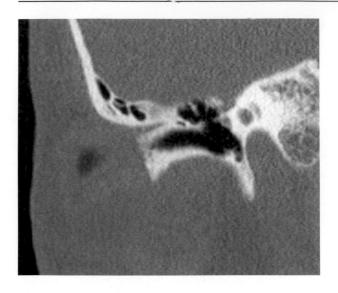

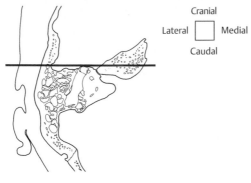

Cranial

Lateral ☐ Medial

Caudal

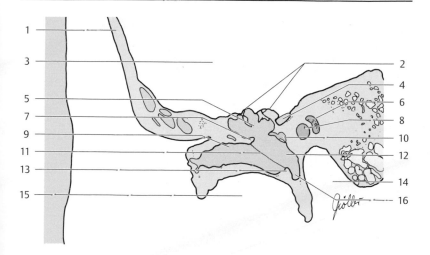

1 Temporal bone
2 Tegmen tympani
3 Middle cranial fossa
4 Geniculate ganglion
5 Epitympanum
6 Cochlea (first turn)
7 Scutum
8 Cochlea (second turn)
9 External acoustic meatus
10 Tensor tympani muscle
11 Tympanic membrane
12 Mesotympanum
13 Tympanic ring, anterior part
14 Internal carotid artery,
   petrous part
15 Temporomandibular joint
16 Hypotympanum

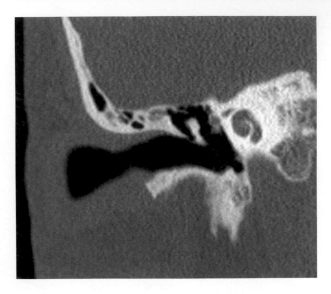

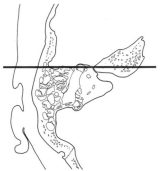

Cranial

Lateral ☐ Medial

Caudal

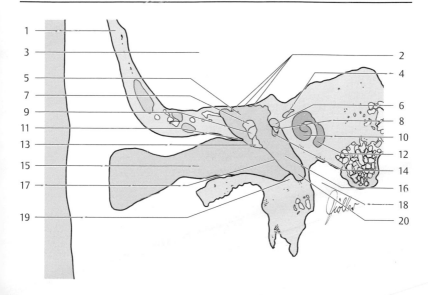

1 Temporal bone
2 Tegmen tympani
3 Middle cranial fossa
4 Facial nerve (cranial nerve VII), labyrinthine segment
5 Epitympanum
6 Facial nerve (cranial nerve VII), anterior tympanic segment
7 Incus (body)
8 Processus cochleariformis
9 Malleus (head)
10 Cochlea (second turn)
11 Scutum
12 Cochlea (first turn)
13 Malleus (manubrium)
14 Tensor tympani muscle (tendon)
15 External acoustic meatus
16 Mesotympanum
17 Tympanic membrane
18 Internal carotid artery, petrous part
19 Tympanic ring
20 Hypotympanum

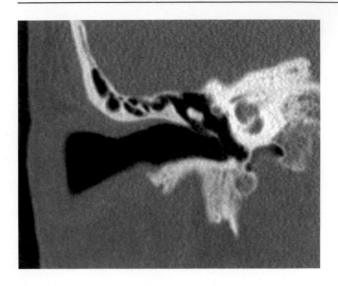

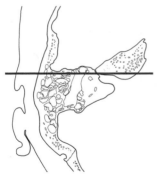

Cranial

Lateral ☐ Medial

Caudal

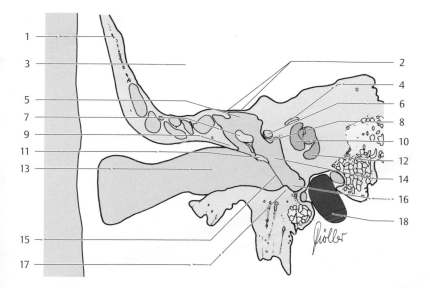

1 Temporal bone
2 Tegmen tympani
3 Middle cranial fossa
4 Facial nerve (cranial nerve VII),
  labyrinthine segment
5 Epitympanum
6 Facial nerve (VII), anterior
  tympanic segment
7 Incus (body)
8 Processus cochleariformis
9 Scutum

10 Cochlea (second turn)
11 Malleus (manubrium)
12 Cochlea (first turn)
13 External acoustic meatus
14 Mesotympanum
15 Tympanic membrane
16 Hypotympanum
17 Tympanic ring
18 Internal carotid artery, petrous
   part

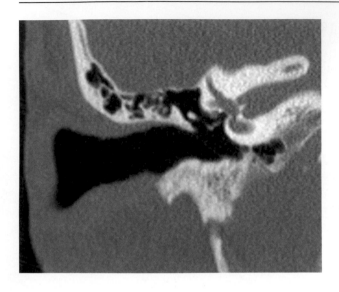

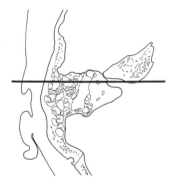

Cranial

Lateral ☐ Medial

Caudal

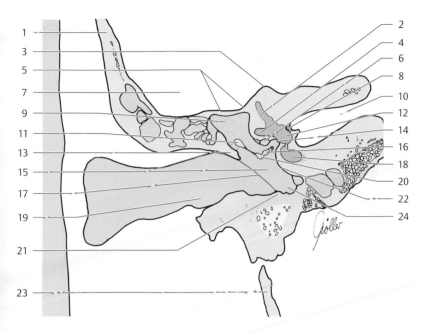

1 Temporal bone	13 Scutum
2 Superior semicircular canal	14 Oval window
3 Arcuate eminence	15 Mesotympanum
4 Lateral semicircular canal	16 Stapes
5 Tegmen tympani	17 Tympanic membrane
6 Facial nerve (cranial nerve VII) posterior genu	18 Cochlea (spiral canal, basal)
7 Middle cranial fossa	19 External acoustic meatus
8 Facial nerve (VII), labyrinthine segment	20 Incus (long crus)
9 Epitympanum	21 Tympanic ring
10 Internal acoustic meatus	22 Promontory through spiral canal (basal) of cochlea
11 Incus (short crus)	23 Styloid process
12 Utricle	24 Hypotympanum

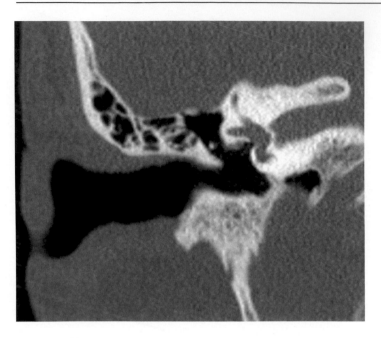

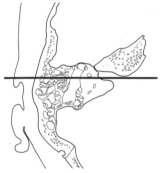

Cranial

Lateral ⬜ Medial

Caudal

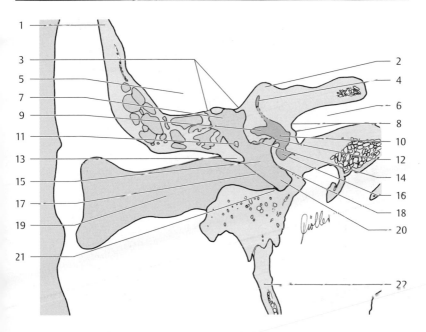

1 Temporal bone
2 Arcuate eminence
3 Tegmen tympani
4 Superior semicircular canal
5 Middle cranial fossa
6 Internal acoustic meatus
7 Epitympanum
8 Fundus of internal acoustic meatus and transverse crest
9 Lateral semicircular canal
10 Vestibule
11 Incus (short crus)
12 Oval window
13 Scutum
14 Facial nerve (VII) in facial nerve canal
15 Mesotympanum
16 Cochlea (spiral canal, basal)
17 Tympanic membrane
18 Promontory through spiral canal (basal) of cochlea
19 External acoustic meatus
20 Hypotympanum
21 Tympanic ring
22 Styloid process

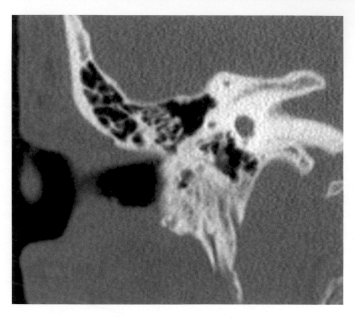

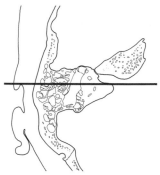

Cranial

Lateral ☐ Medial

Caudal

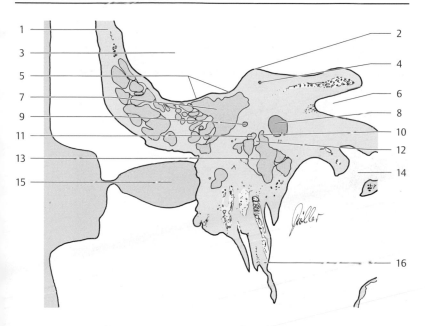

1 Temporal bone
2 Arcuate eminence
3 Middle cranial fossa
4 Superior semicircular canal
5 Tegmen tympani
6 Internal acoustic meatus
7 Mastoid antrum
8 Vestibule
9 Lateral semicircular canal
10 Tympanic sinus
11 Facial nerve (VII, posterior genu)
12 Pyramidal eminence
13 Mesotympanum
14 Hypoglossal canal
15 External acoustic meatus
16 Styloid process

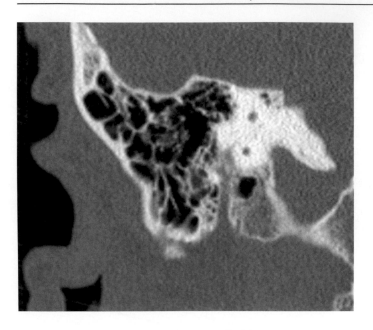

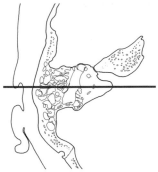

Cranial

Lateral ▢ Medial

Caudal

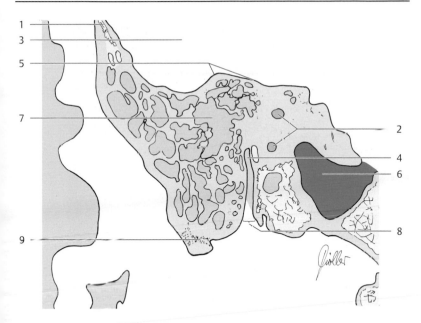

1 Temporal bone
2 Posterior semicircular canal
3 Middle cranial fossa
4 Facial nerve (VII), mastoid
   segment
5 Mastoid tegmen
6 Jugular foramen
7 Mastoid antrum
8 Stylomastoid foramen
9 Mastoid process

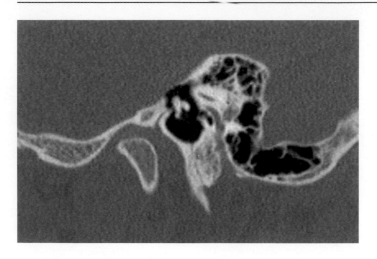

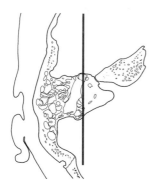

Cranial

Frontal ☐ Occipital

Caudal

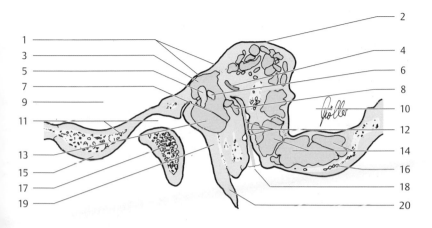

1 Tegmen tympani
2 Petrous part of temporal bone
(superior margin)
3 Epitympanic recess (anterior)
4 Lateral semicircular canal
5 Malleus (head)
6 Incus
7 Tympanic membrane
8 Chorda tympani
9 Middle cranial fossa
10 Posterior cranial fossa
11 Temporal bone and mandibular fossa (temporomandibular
joint)

12 Facial nerve (VII) in facial
nerve canal
13 External acoustic meatus
14 Mastoid cells
15 Articular tubercle (of temporal
bone)
16 Temporal bone, petrous part
17 Head of mandible
18 Stylomastoid foramen
19 Temporal bone, tympanic part
20 Styloid process

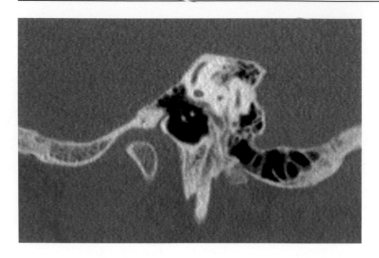

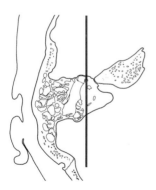

Cranial

Frontal ☐ Occipital

Caudal

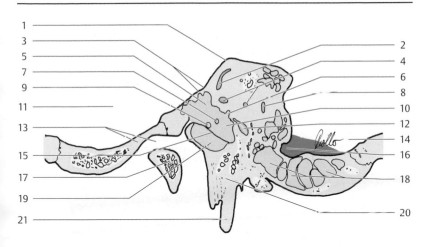

1 Petrous part of temporal bone (superior margin)
2 Superior semicircular canal
3 Tegmen tympani
4 Lateral semicircular canal
5 Epitympanum
6 Vestibule
7 Incus
8 Posterior semicircular canal
9 Facial nerve (VII), anterior tympanic segment
10 Mesotympanum
11 Middle cranial fossa
12 Facial nerve canal (VII)
13 Temporal bone and mandibular fossa (temporomandibular joint)
14 Posterior cranial fossa
15 Tympanic membrane
16 Sigmoid sinus
17 Head of mandible
18 Mastoid cells
19 External acoustic meatus
20 Temporal bone, petrous part
21 Styloid process

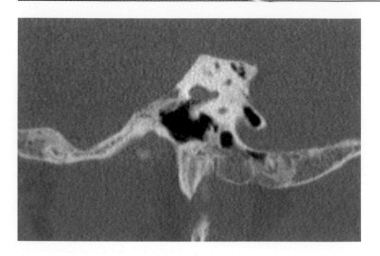

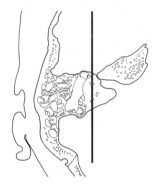

Cranial

Frontal ☐ Occipital

Caudal

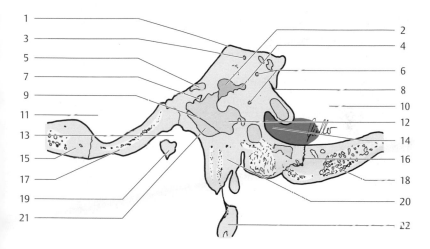

1 Petrous part of temporal bone (superior margin)
2 Vestibule
3 Superior semicircular canal
4 Lateral semicircular canal
5 Facial nerve (VII), geniculate ganglion
6 Posterior semicircular canal
7 Tensor tympani muscle
8 External opening of vestibular aqueduct
9 Tympanic membrane
10 Posterior cranial fossa
11 Middle cranial fossa
12 Hypotympanum
13 Mandibular fossa (temporomandibular joint)
14 Sigmoid sinus
15 Sphenoid (greater wing)
16 Occipitomastoid suture
17 Temporal bone
18 Occipital bone
19 Head of mandible
20 Temporal bone, petrous part
21 External acoustic meatus
22 Styloid process

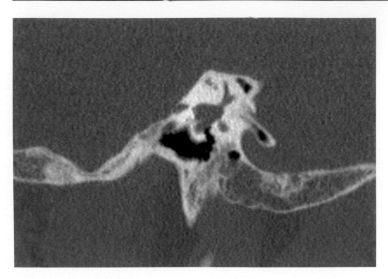

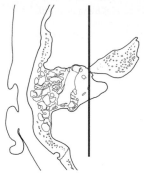

Cranial

Frontal ☐ Occipital

Caudal

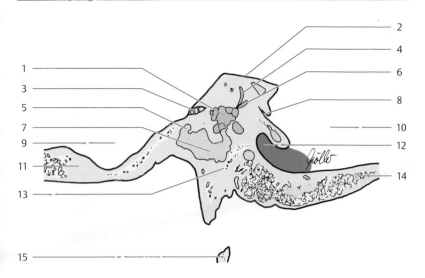

1 Vestibule
2 Petrous part of temporal bone
(superior margin)
3 Facial nerve canal (VII)
4 Superior semicircular canal
5 Tensor tympani muscle
6 Posterior semicircular canal
7 Hypotympanum

8 External opening of vestibular
aqueduct
9 Middle cranial fossa
10 Posterior cranial fossa
11 Sphenoid (greater wing)
12 Internal jugular vein (bulb)
13 Temporal bone, petrous part
14 Occipital bone
15 Styloid process

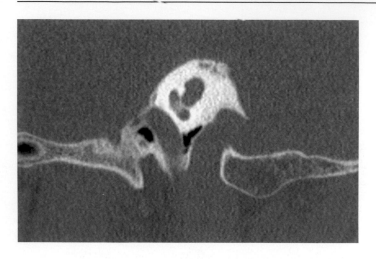

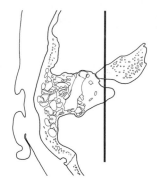

Cranial

Frontal ☐ Occipital

Caudal

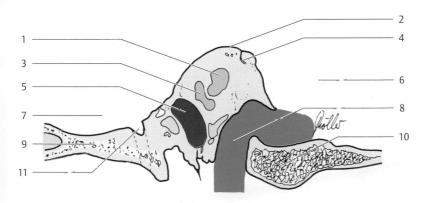

1 Internal acoustic meatus
2 Petrous part of temporal bone (superior margin)
3 Cochlea (first turn)
4 Vestibular aqueduct
5 Internal carotid artery in carotid canal
6 Posterior cranial fossa
7 Middle cranial fossa
8 Jugular foramen with internal jugular vein (bulb)
9 Sphenoid (greater wing)
10 Occipital bone
11 Foramen spinosum

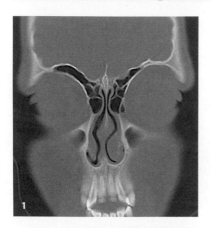

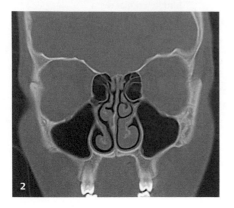

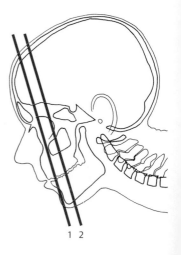

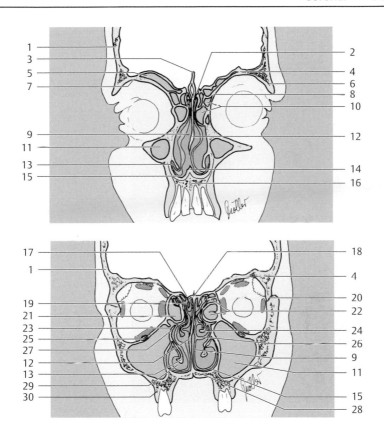

1 Frontal bone
2 Cribriform plate
3 Crista galli
4 Roof of orbit
5 Frontal sinus
6 Zygomatic process
7 Supraorbital notch
8 Orbital plate
9 Nasal cavity
10 Anterior ethmoidal cells
11 Maxillary sinus
12 Nasal septum
13 Inferior nasal concha
14 Vomer
15 Inferior nasal meatus
16 Alveolar process of maxilla
17 Ethmoidal notch
18 Ethmoidal bone (cribriform plate)
19 Superior nasal concha
20 Frontozygomatic suture
21 Orbital plate of ethmoidal labyrinth
22 Ethmoidal cells (middle)
23 Maxillary hiatus
24 Middle nasal concha
25 Infraorbital foramen
26 Middle nasal meatus
27 Uncinate process
28 Hard palate
29 Inferior nasal concha
30 Maxilla (alveolar process)

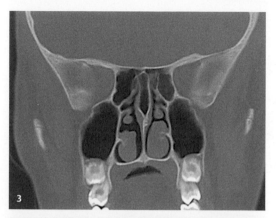

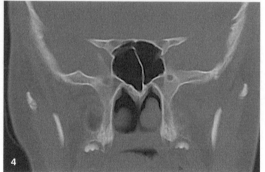

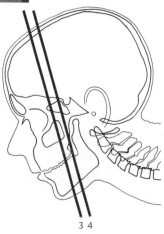

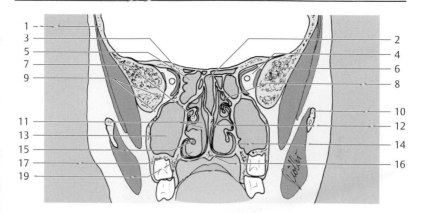

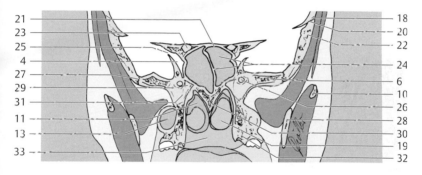

1 Frontal bone	18 Parietal bone
2 Sphenoidal sinus (recess)	19 Inferior nasal concha
3 Sphenoidal bone (lesser wing)	(cavernous body)
4 Infundibulum of orbit	20 Squamous suture
5 Ethmoidal cells (posterior)	21 Sphenoidal bone (roof of
6 Sphenoidal bone (greater wing)	splenoidal sinus)
7 Middle nasal concha	22 Temporal bone (squamous part)
8 Superior nasal concha	23 Optic canal
9 Inferior orbital fissure	24 Sphenoidal sinus with septum
10 Zygomatic bone	25 Superior orbital fissure
11 Nasal cavity (common nasal	26 Foramen rotundum of
meatus)	sphenoidal bone
12 Nasal septum (perpendicular	27 Sphenosquamous suture
palate)	28 Mandible (body and ramus)
13 Maxillary sinus	29 Pterygoid canal
14 Inferior nasal meatus	30 Ethmoidal bone (nasal septum)
15 Inferior nasal concha	31 Pterygopalatine fossa
16 Palatine bone (horizontal plane)	32 Pterygoid process
17 Maxilla (alveolar process)	33 Soft palate

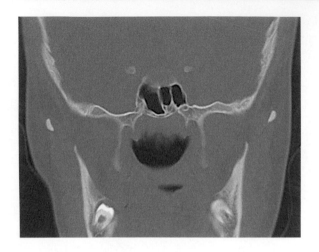

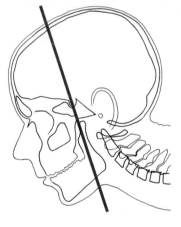

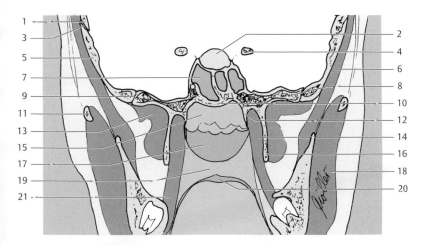

1 Parietal bone
2 Sella turcica
3 Squamous suture
4 Anterior clinoid process
  (sphenoidal bone)
5 Temporal bone (squamous
  part)
6 Temporal muscle
7 Sphenoidal sinus
8 Temporal bone (with articular
  tubercle)
9 Sphenosquamous suture
10 Sphenoidal bone
11 Zygomatic arch
12 Pterygoid process (medial plate)
13 Lateral pterygoid muscle
14 Pterygoid fossa
15 Pharyngeal tonsil
16 Pterygoid process (lateral plate)
17 Nasopharynx
18 Masseter muscle
19 Soft palate
20 Oropharynx (isthmus of fauces)
21 Medial pterygoid muscle

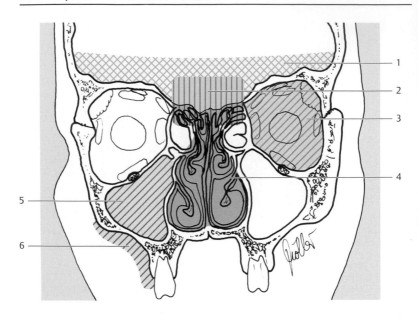

▨	1 Anterior cranial fossa
▥	2 Base of the nose
▨	3 Orbital cavity
▦	4 Nasal cavity
▨	5 Maxillary sinus
▨	6 Buccal space

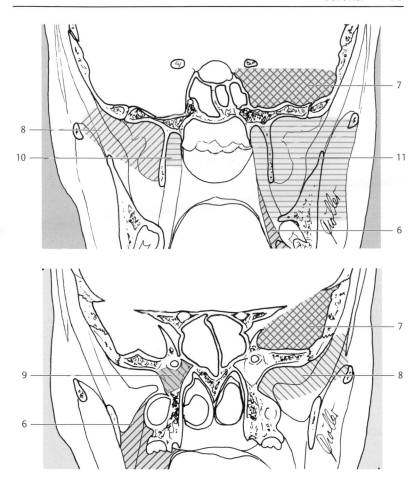

6 Buccal space
7 Middle cranial fossa
8 Infratemporal fossa
9 Pterygopalatine fossa
10 Pterygoid fossa
11 Masticatory space

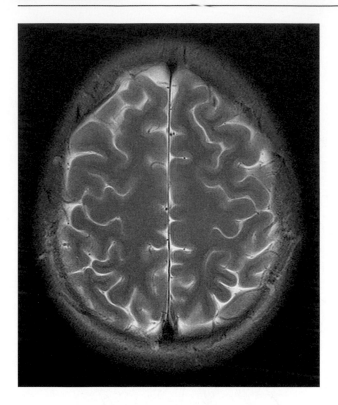

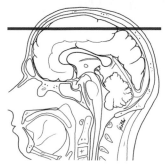

Frontal lobe
Parietal lobe

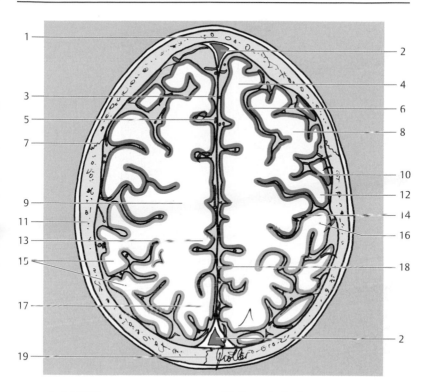

1   Frontal bone
2   Superior sagittal sinus
3   Longitudinal cerebral fissure
4   Superior frontal gyrus
5   Supratrochlear artery (postero-
    medial)
6   Superior frontal sulcus
7   Coronal suture
8   Middle frontal gyrus
9   Cerebral white matter
    (semioval center)

10 Precentral sulcus
11 Parietal bone
12 Precentral gyrus
13 Paracentral lobule
14 Central sulcus
15 Superior parietal lobule
16 Postcentral gyrus
17 Precuneus
18 Falx cerebri
19 Sagittal suture

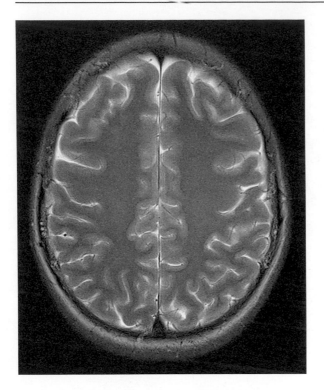

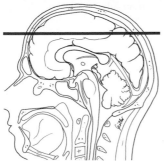

Frontal lobe
Parietal lobe
Occipital lobe

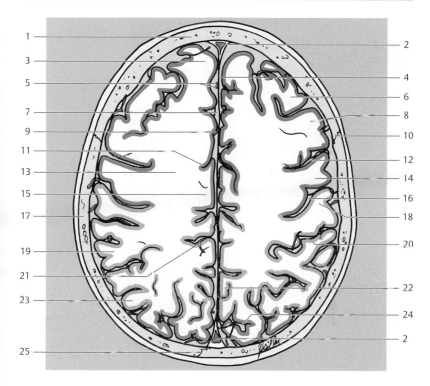

1 Frontal bone
2 Superior sagittal sinus
3 Superior frontal gyrus
4 Falx cerebri
5 Supratrochlear artery
   (mediomedial)
6 Middle frontal gyrus
7 Longitudinal cerebral fissure
8 Inferior frontal gyrus
9 Callosomarginal artery
10 Coronal suture
11 Cingulate sulcus
12 Precentral sulcus
13 Cerebral white matter
   (semioval center)
14 Precentral gyrus
15 Cingulate gyrus and cingulum
16 Central sulcus (fissure of Rolando)
17 Parietal bone
18 Postcentral gyrus
19 Supramarginal gyrus
20 Postcentral sulcus
21 Paracentral branches of
   callosomarginal artery
22 Precuneus
23 Angular gyrus
24 Parieto-occipital sulcus
25 Sagittal suture

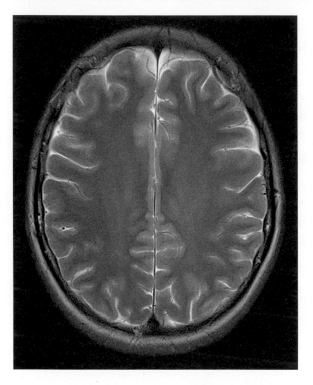

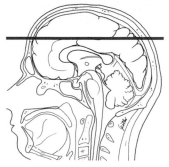

Frontal lobe
Parietal lobe
Occipital lobe

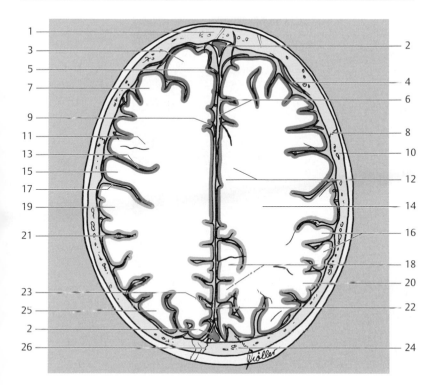

1 Frontal bone
2 Superior sagittal sinus
3 Superior frontal gyrus
4 Superior cerebral vein
5 Supratrochlear (mediomedial)
   artery
6 Longitudinal cerebral fissure
7 Middle frontal gyrus
8 Coronal suture
9 Callosomarginal artery
10 Parietal bone
11 Inferior frontal gyrus
12 Cingulate gyrus and cingulum
13 Precentral sulcus

14 Cerebral white matter
   (semioval center)
15 Precentral gyrus
16 Supramarginal gyrus
17 Central sulcus
18 Precuneus
19 Postcentral gyrus
20 Angular gyrus
21 Postcentral sulcus
22 Falx cerebri
23 Parieto-occipital sulcus
24 Occipital bone
25 Occipital gyri
26 Lambdoid suture

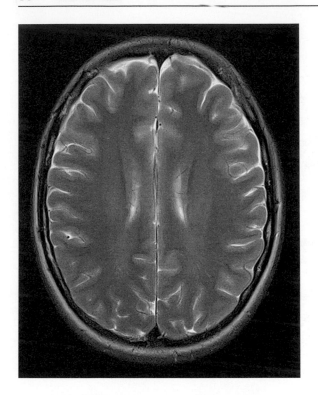

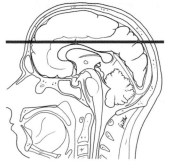

Frontal lobe
Parietal lobe
Occipital lobe

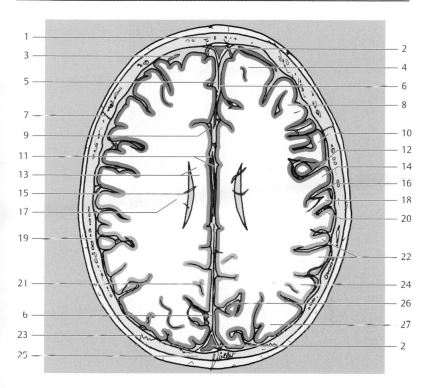

1 Frontal bone	15 Lateral ventricle (central part)
2 Superior sagittal sinus	16 Central sulcus
3 Superior cerebral vein	17 Corona radiata
4 Superior frontal gyrus	18 Postcentral gyrus
5 Longitudinal cerebral fissure	19 Parietal bone
6 Falx cerebri	20 Postcentral sulcus
7 Coronal suture	21 Precuneus
8 Middle frontal gyrus	22 Supramarginal gyrus
9 Callosomarginal artery	23 Lambdoid suture
10 Inferior frontal gyrus	24 Angular gyrus
11 Pericallosal artery	25 Occipital bone
12 Precentral sulcus	26 Parieto-occipital sulcus
13 Cingulate gyrus and cingulum	27 Occipital gyri
14 Precentral gyrus	

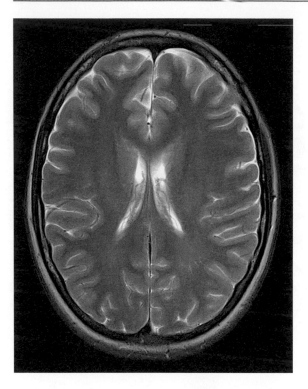

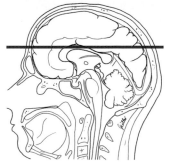

Frontal lobe
Parietal lobe
Occipital lobe

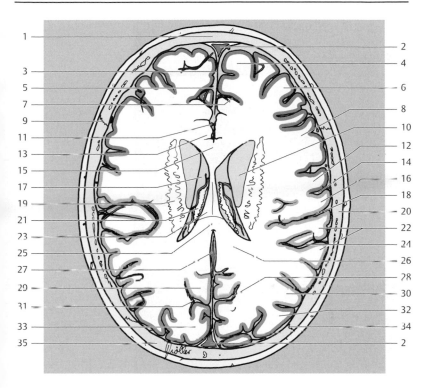

1 Frontal bone
2 Superior sagittal sinus
3 Falx cerebri
4 Superior frontal gyrus
5 Longitudinal cerebral fissure
6 Middle frontal gyrus
7 Cingulate sulcus
8 Inferior frontal gyrus
9 Coronal suture
10 Head of caudate nucleus
11 Pericallosal artery
12 Precentral gyrus
13 Cingulate gyrus
14 Central sulcus
15 Corpus callosum (genu)
16 Postcentral gyrus
17 Lateral ventricle
18 Lateral sulcus

19 Corona radiata
20 Parietal bone
21 Choroid plexus
22 Supramarginal gyrus
23 Fornix
24 Lateral sulcus (posterior ramus)
25 Corpus callosum, splenium
26 Major forceps (occipital forceps)
27 Inferior sagittal sinus
28 Parieto-occipital sulcus
29 Precuneus
30 Angular gyrus
31 Parieto-occipital artery
32 Occipital gyri
33 Cuneus
34 Lambdoid suture
35 Occipital bone

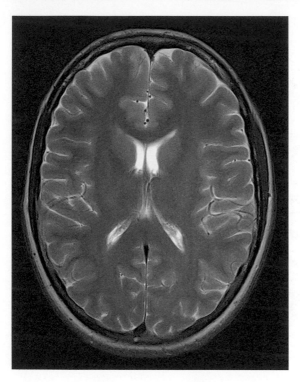

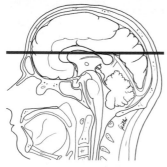

Frontal lobe
Temporal lobe
Parietal lobe
Occipital lobe

1 Frontal bone
2 Superior sagittal sinus
3 Falx cerebri
4 Superior frontal gyrus
5 Cingulate sulcus
6 Cingulate gyrus

7 Pericallosal artery
8 Middle frontal gyrus
9 Corpus callosum (genu)
10 Lateral ventricle (frontal horn)
11 Head of caudate nucleus
12 Inferior frontal gyrus ►

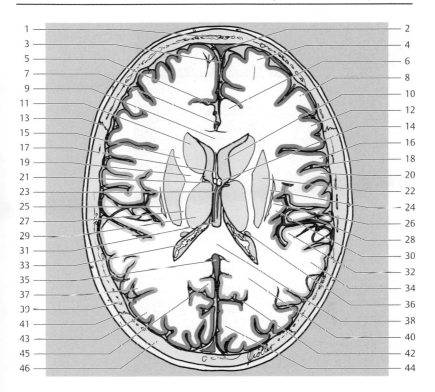

13 Coronal suture
14 Fornix (column)
15 Internal capsule (anterior limb)
16 Precentral gyrus
17 Cave of septum pellucidum
18 Central sulcus
19 Internal capsule (genu)
20 Postcentral gyrus
21 Interventricular foramen
    (foramen of Monro)
22 Putamen
23 Internal cerebral vein
24 External capsule
25 Claustrum
26 Extreme capsule
27 Internal capsule (posterior
    limb)
28 Lateral sulcus
29 Thalamus

30 Insula
31 Third ventricle (suprapineal recess)
32 Transverse temporal gyrus
33 Choroid plexus in trigone of posterior
    horn of lateral ventricle
34 Superior temporal gyrus
35 Great cerebral vein
36 Tail of caudate nucleus
37 Angular gyrus
38 Corpus callosum, splenium
39 Parietal bone
40 Major forceps (occipital forceps)
41 Lambdoid suture
42 Parieto-occipital sulcus
43 Occipital gyri
44 Cuneus
45 Precuneus
46 Occipital bone

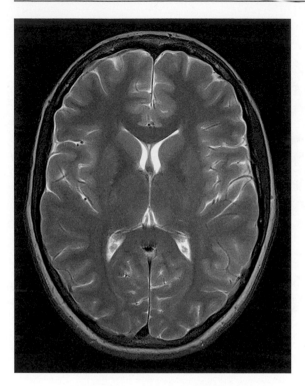

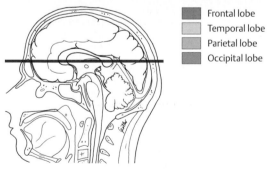

■ Frontal lobe
■ Temporal lobe
■ Parietal lobe
■ Occipital lobe

1 Frontal bone	6 Middle frontal gyrus
2 Superior sagittal sinus	7 Pericallosal artery
3 Falx cerebri	8 Coronal suture
4 Superior frontal gyrus	9 Corpus callosum (genu)
5 Cingulate gyrus	10 Inferior frontal gyrus

▶

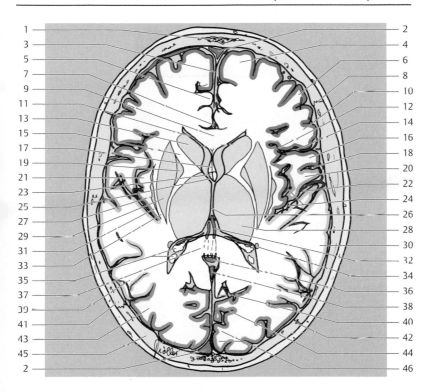

11 Lateral ventricle (frontal horn)
12 Circular sulcus of insula
13 Head of caudate nucleus
14 Lateral sulcus
15 Internal capsule (anterior limb)
16 Precentral gyrus
17 Cave of septum pellucidum
18 Central sulcus
19 Globus pallidus
20 Postcentral gyrus
21 Insula
22 Cistern of lateral cerebral fossa
   (insular cistern)
23 Fornix (column)
24 Insular arteries
25 Interventricular foramen
   (foramen of Monro)
26 Third ventricle
27 Claustrum
28 Thalamus

29 Putamen
30 Superior temporal gyrus
31 Extreme capsule
32 Internal cerebral vein
33 External capsule
34 Tail of caudate nucleus
35 Choroid plexus in trigone of posterior
   horn of lateral ventricle
36 Great cerebral vein
37 Corpus callosum, splenium
38 Straight sinus
39 Middle temporal gyrus
40 Parieto-occipital sulcus
41 Parietal bone
42 Lambdoid suture
43 Occipital gyri
44 Cuneus
45 Occipital bone
46 Striate cortex

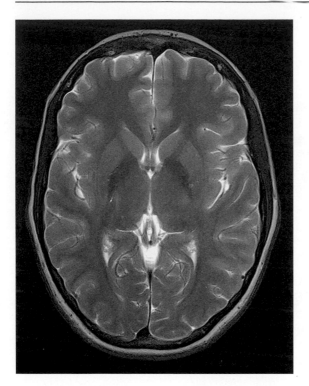

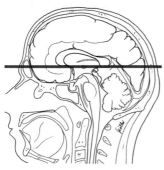

Frontal lobe
Temporal lobe
Parietal lobe
Occipital lobe

1 Frontal bone
2 Superior sagittal sinus
3 Falx cerebri
4 Superior frontal gyrus
5 Cingulate gyrus

6 Middle frontal gyrus
7 Anterior cerebral artery
8 Coronal suture
9 Lateral ventricle
   (frontal horn)

▶

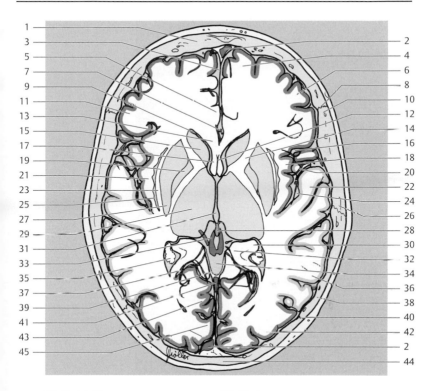

10 Parietal bone
11 Inferior frontal gyrus
12 Cave of septum pellucidum
13 Corpus callosum
14 Internal capsule (anterior limb)
15 Head of caudate nucleus
16 Lateral sulcus
17 Fornix
18 Insula
19 Pallidum
20 Insular arteries
21 Extreme capsule
22 Superior temporal gyrus
23 External capsule
24 Insular cistern
25 Claustrum
26 Temporal bone
27 Putamen
28 Epiphysis of cerebrum

29 Thalamus
30 Hippocampus
31 Third ventricle
32 Uncus of parahippocampal gyrus
33 Internal cerebral vein and great
    cerebral vein
34 Superior cerebellar cistern
35 Choroid plexus in trigone of posterior
    horn of lateral ventricle
36 Middle temporal gyrus
37 Parieto-occipital artery
38 Parietal bone
39 Tentorium cerebelli
40 Lambdoid suture
41 Straight sinus
42 Occipital gyri
43 Cuneus
44 Occipital bone
45 Striate cortex

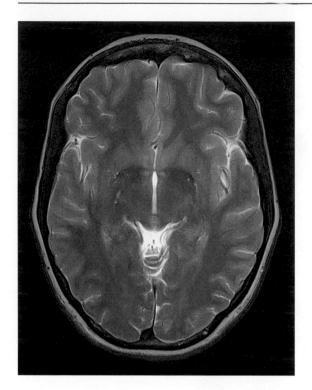

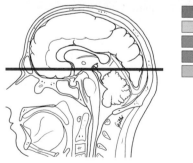

Frontal lobe
Temporal lobe
Occipital lobe
Cerebellum
Mesencephalon

1 Frontal bone
2 Superior frontal gyrus
3 Cingulate gyrus
4 Falx cerebri
5 Anterior cerebral artery

6   Middle frontal gyrus
7   Inferior frontal gyrus
8   Head of caudate nucleus
9   Lateral sulcus
10 Internal capsule (anterior limb)

▶

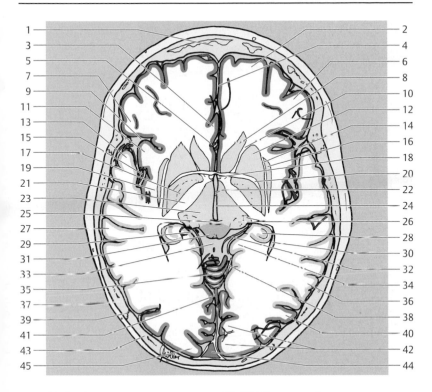

11 Insula
12 Putamen
13 Superior temporal gyrus
14 External capsule
15 Insular arteries
16 Claustrum
17 Globus pallidus (lateral and medial segments)
18 Fornix
19 Extreme capsule
20 Anterior commissure
21 Internal capsule (posterior limb)
22 Interthalamic adhesion
23 Thalamus
24 Third ventricle
25 Posterior commissure
26 Medial and lateral geniculate body

27 Middle temporal gyrus
28 Hippocampus
29 Ambient cistern
30 Lateral ventricle (temporal horn)
31 Inferior colliculus
32 Basal vein
33 Quadrigeminal cistern
34 Uncus of parahippocampal gyrus
35 Vermis of superior cerebellar lobe
36 Inferior temporal gyrus
37 Temporal bone
38 Tentorium cerebelli
39 Lambdoid suture
40 Occipital gyri
41 Straight sinus
42 Striate cortex
43 Occipital bone
44 Superior sagittal sinus
45 Occipital pole

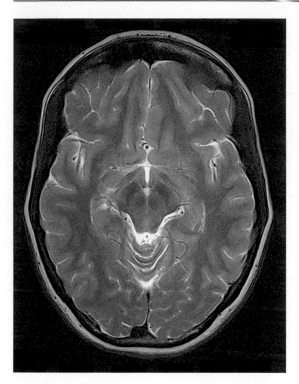

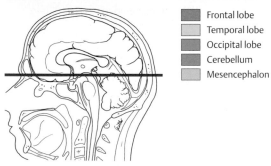

Frontal lobe
Temporal lobe
Occipital lobe
Cerebellum
Mesencephalon

1 Frontal sinus
2 Superior frontal gyrus
3 Frontal bone
4 Falx cerebri
5 Optic tract

6 Cingulate gyrus
7 Circular sulcus of insula
8 Middle frontal gyrus
9 Lateral sulcus
10 Anterior cerebral artery

▶

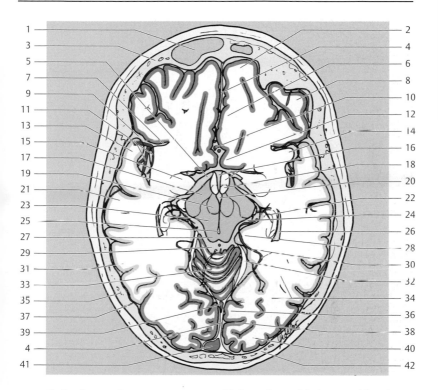

11 Insular arteries
12 Subcallosal cortex
13 Superior temporal gyrus
14 Insula
15 Amygdaloid body
16 Third ventricle (optic recess) and hypothalamus
17 Cerebral peduncle
18 Mammillary body
19 Red nucleus
20 Interpeduncular fossa
21 Middle temporal gyrus
22 Hippocampus
23 Tegmentum of midbrain
24 Ambient cistern
25 Aqueduct of mesencephalon
26 Lateral ventricle (temporal horn)
27 Inferior colliculus
28 Uncus of parahippocampal gyrus
29 Quadrigeminal cistern
30 Posterior cerebral artery
31 Inferior temporal gyrus
32 Tentorium cerebelli
33 Anterior cerebellar lobule (vermis)
34 Optic radiation
35 Temporal bone
36 Striate cortex
37 Lambdoid suture
38 Calcarine sulcus
39 Straight sinus
40 Occipital pole
41 Superior sagittal sinus
42 Occipital bone

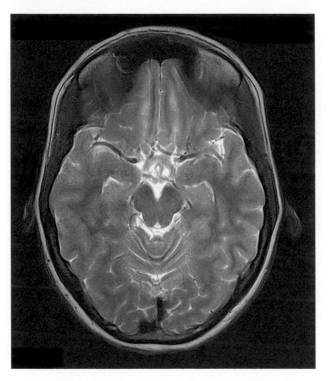

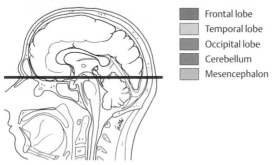

Frontal lobe
Temporal lobe
Occipital lobe
Cerebellum
Mesencephalon

1 Frontal sinus
2 Frontal bone
3 Falx cerebri
4 Orbital roof
5 Straight gyrus

6 Orbital gyrus
7 Sphenoidal bone
8 Temporal muscle
9 Optic chiasm
10 Olfactory sulcus

▶

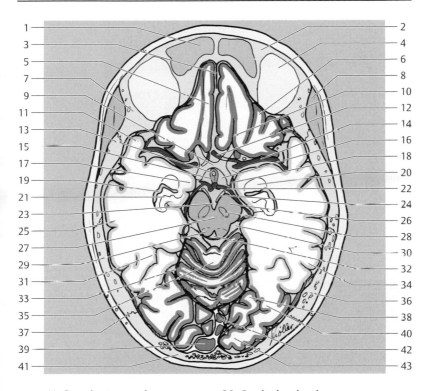

11 Superior temporal gyrus	26 Cerebral peduncle
12 Anterior cerebral artery	27 Tegmentum of midbrain
13 Infundibular recess	28 Substantia nigra
14 Middle cerebral artery	29 Inferior colliculus
15 Hypothalamus	30 Ambient cistern
16 Chiasmatic cistern	31 Collateral sulcus
17 Uncus of parahippocampal gyrus	32 Aqueduct of midbrain
18 Posterior communicating artery	33 Tentorium cerebelli
19 Lateral ventricle (temporal horn)	34 Inferior temporal gyrus
20 Amygdaloid body	35 Anterior cerebellar lobe
21 Hippocampus	36 Temporal bone
22 Posterior cerebral artery	37 Lambdoid suture
23 Interpeduncular cistern	38 Medial occipitotemporal gyrus
24 Oculomotor nerve (III)	39 Superior sagittal sinus
25 Middle temporal gyrus	40 Lateral occipitotemporal gyrus
	41 Occipital bone
	42 Straight sinus
	43 Occipital gyri

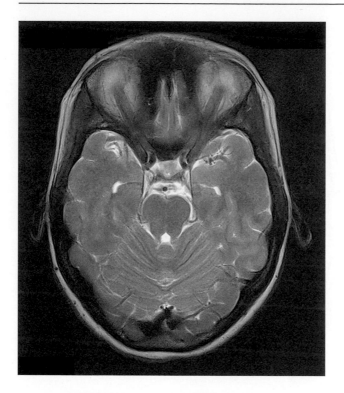

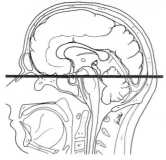

Temporal lobe
Occipital lobe
Cerebellum
Mesencephalon
Pons

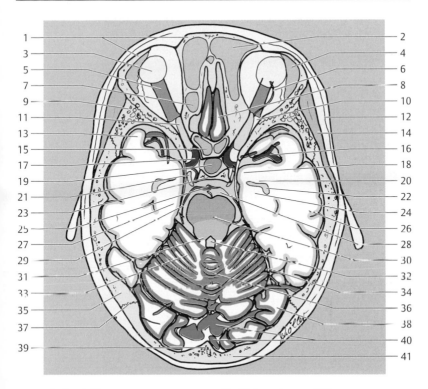

1 Frontal bone	21 Abducent nerve (VI)
2 Frontal sinus	22 Lateral ventricle (temporal horn)
3 Eyeball	23 Dorsum sellae
4 Lacrimal gland	24 Hippocampus
5 Superior rectus muscle	25 Basilar artery
6 Ophthalmic vein	26 Middle temporal gyrus
7 Ethmoidal cells	27 Parahippocampal gyrus
8 Straight gyrus	28 Prepontine cistern
9 Sphenoidal bone	29 Posterior cerebral artery
10 Superior orbital fissure	30 Pons
11 Optic nerve (II)	31 Superior cerebellar peduncle
12 Temporoparietal muscle	32 Fourth ventricle
13 Superior temporal gyrus	33 Anterior lobe of cerebellum
14 Temporal muscle	34 Tentorium cerebelli
15 Sphenoidal sinus	35 Temporal bone
16 Middle cerebral artery	36 Vermis of cerebellum
17 Internal carotid artery	37 Lambdoid suture
18 Uncus of parahippocampal gyrus	38 Occipital gyri
19 Pituitary gland	39 Internal occipital protuberance
20 Amygdaloid body	40 Confluence of sinuses
	41 Occipital bone

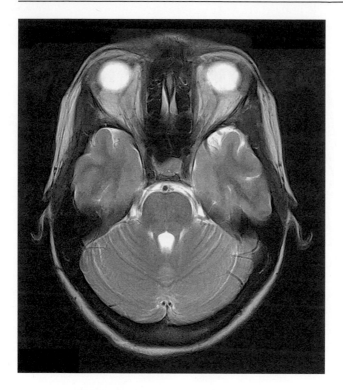

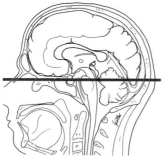

Temporal lobe
Cerebellum
Pons

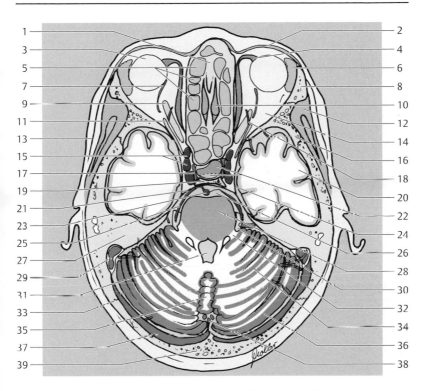

1 Ethmoidal bone
2 Orbicularis oris muscle and occipitofrontal muscle
3 Eyeball
4 Medial rectus muscle
5 Ethmoidal cells
6 Lacrimal gland
7 Superior ophthalmic vein
8 Zygomatic bone
9 Optic nerve (II)
10 Olfactory bulb
11 Oculomotor (III) and abducent (VI) nerves
12 Temporal muscle
13 Temporoparietal muscle
14 Retro-orbital fatty tissue
15 Internal carotid artery
16 Sphenoidal bone
17 Cavernous sinus
18 Ophthalmic artery
19 Dorsum sellae

20 Inferior temporal gyrus
21 Posterior petroclinoid ligament
22 Pituitary gland (neurohypophysis and adenohypophysis)
23 Basilar artery
24 Anterior petroclinoid ligament
25 Posterior cerebral artery
26 Prepontine cistern
27 Petrous part of temporal bone
28 Pons
29 Sigmoid sinus
30 Trigeminal nerve (V)
31 Fourth ventricle
32 Middle cerebellar peduncle
33 Lambdoid suture
34 Anterior lobe of cerebellum
35 Vermis of cerebellum
36 Posterior lobe of cerebellum
37 Transverse sinus
38 Occipital sinus
39 Occipital bone

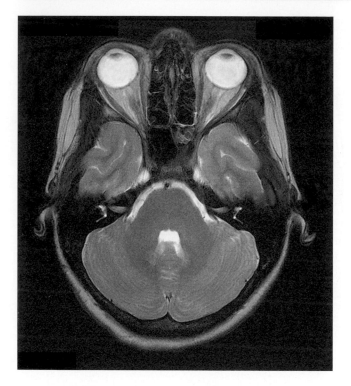

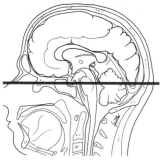

Temporal lobe
Cerebellum
Pons

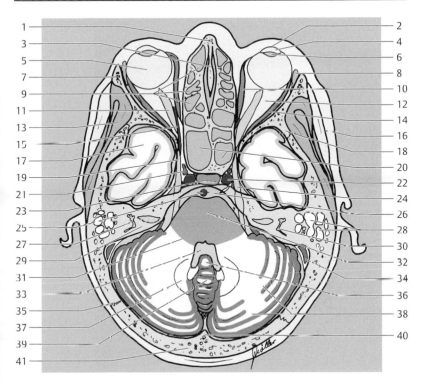

1 Nasal bone	22 Internal carotid artery
2 Cornea	23 Pituitary gland
3 Nasal septum	24 Trigeminal ganglion
4 Anterior chamber of eyeball	25 Basilar artery
5 Eyeball	26 Prepontine cistern
6 Lens	27 Cochlea
7 Zygomatic bone	28 Mastoid cells
8 Lacrimal gland	29 Petrous part of temporal bone
9 Ethmoidal cells	30 Semicircular canal
10 Medial rectus muscle	31 Middle cerebellar peduncle
11 Optic nerve (II)	32 Pons
12 Retro-orbital fatty tissue	33 Fourth ventricle
13 Temporal muscle	34 Sigmoid sinus
14 Lateral rectus muscle	35 Lambdoid suture
15 Ophthalmic artery	36 Uvula of vermis
16 Temporoparietal muscle	37 Dentate nucleus
17 Temporal lobe (temporal pole)	38 Posterior lobe of cerebellum
18 Sphenoidal bone	39 Vermis of cerebellum
19 Oculomotor nerve (III)	40 Internal occipital protuberance
20 Sphenoidal sinus	41 Occipital bone
21 Cavernous sinus	

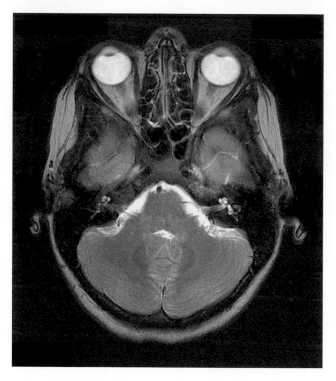

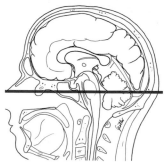

Temporal lobe
Cerebellum
Pons

1 Nasal bone
2 Cornea
3 Ethmoidal cells
4 Anterior chamber of eyeball
5 Eyeball

6 Lens
7 Zygomatic bone
8 Medial rectus muscle
9 Optic nerve (II)
10 Lateral rectus muscle

►

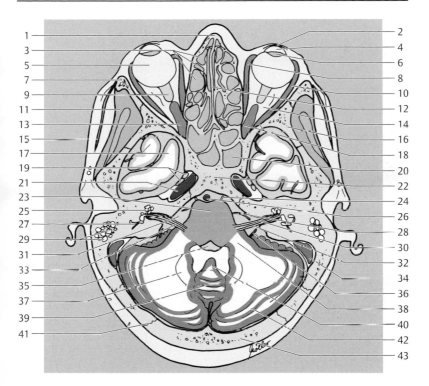

11 Temporal muscle	27 Posterior semicircular canal
12 Nasal septum	28 Superior cerebellar artery
13 Superior rectus muscle and	29 Mastoid cells
levator palpebrae superioris	30 Facial nerve (VII) and intermediate
muscle	nerve
14 Retro-orbital fatty tissue	31 Internal acoustic meatus
15 Temporoparietal muscle	32 Vestibulocochlear (auditory)
16 Sphenoidal bone	nerve (VIII)
17 Temporal pole	33 Pontocerebellar cistern
18 Superior orbital fissure	34 Sigmoid sinus
19 Maxillary and mandibular	35 Fourth ventricle
nerves	36 Anterior inferior cerebellar artery
20 Sphenoidal sinus	37 Dentate nucleus
21 Internal carotid artery	38 Middle cerebellar peduncle
22 Clivus	39 Vermis of cerebellum
23 Pons	40 Uvula of vermis
24 Abducent nerve (VI)	41 Lambdoid suture
25 Cochlea	42 Caudal lobule of cerebellum
26 Basilar artery	43 Occipital bone

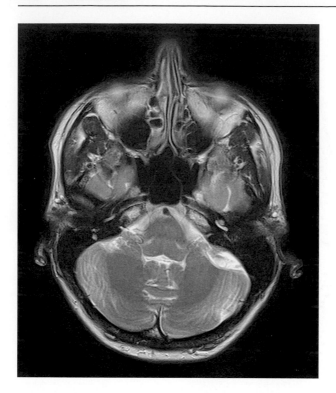

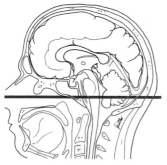

Temporal lobe
Cerebellum
Pons
Medulla oblongata

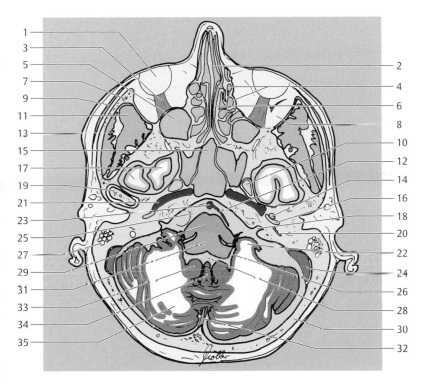

1 Eyeball
2 Nasal septum
3 Inferior rectus muscle
4 Ethmoidal cells
5 Maxillary sinus
6 Nasal sinus
7 Zygomatic bone
8 Retrobulbar fat
9 Orbicularis oris muscle
10 Trigeminal nerve (V)
11 Temporal muscle
12 Anterior inferior cerebellar artery
13 Masseter muscle
14 Cochlea
15 Sphenoidal sinus
16 Vestibule
17 Inferior temporal gyrus
18 Internal acoustic meatus
19 Head of mandible
20 Posterior semicircular canal
21 Internal carotid artery
22 Flocculus
23 Basilar artery
24 Transverse sinus
25 Pontocerebellar cistern
26 Lateral aperture of fourth ventricle (foramen of Luschka)
27 Mastoid cells
28 Fourth ventricle
29 Pons
30 Occipital bone
31 Medulla oblongata
32 Falx cerebelli
33 Tonsil of cerebellum
34 Vermis of cerebellum
35 Cerebellum

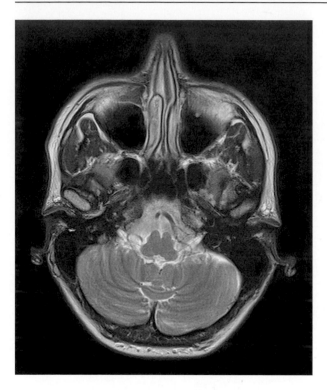

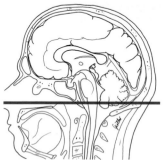

■ Cerebellum
□ Medulla oblongata

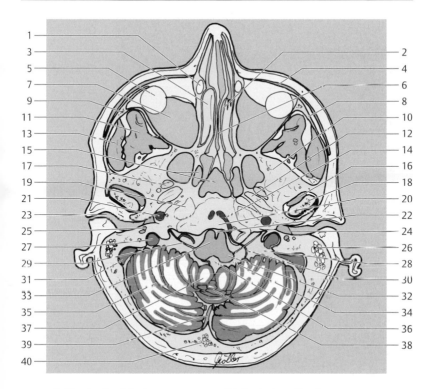

1 Nasolacrimal duct
2 Nasal cavity
3 Nasal concha
4 Orbicularis oris muscle
5 Eyeball
6 Nasal septum
7 Maxillary sinus
8 Sphenoidal bone
9 Zygomatic bone
10 Temporal bone
11 Temporal muscle
12 Pharyngotympanic tube
   (auditory tube)
13 Masseter muscle
14 Vertebral artery
15 Sphenoidal bone
16 Articular disc
17 Trigeminal nerve (V)
18 Head of mandible
19 Foramen lacerum
20 Clivus
21 Internal carotid artery

22 Ventral median fissure
23 External acoustic meatus
24 Tympanic membrane
25 Cochlea
26 Mastoid cells
27 Internal jugular vein
28 Pontocerebellar cistern
29 Glossopharyngeal nerve (IX) and
   vagus nerve (X)
30 Anterior inferior cerebellar artery
31 Sigmoid sinus
32 Medulla oblongata (caudal cerebellar
   peduncle)
33 Medulla oblongata (olivary nucleus)
34 Lateral aperture of fourth ventricle
   (foramen of Luschka)
35 Cerebellum (posterior lobe)
36 Fourth ventricle
37 Tonsil of cerebellum
38 Vermis of cerebellum
39 Falx cerebelli
40 Occipital bone

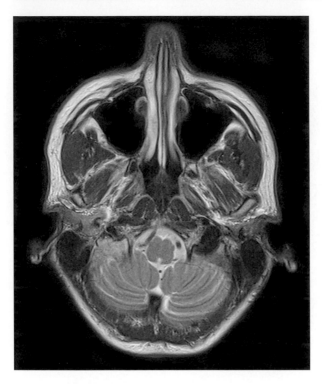

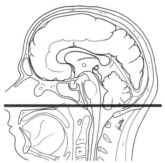

■ Cerebellum
■ Medulla oblongata

1 Nasal bone
2 Nasal septum
3 Superior nasal concha
4 Maxilla (with infra-orbital canal)
5 Levator labii superioris muscle
6 Medial wall of maxillary sinus (with maxillary hiatus)
7 Orbicularis oris muscle
8 Vomer (sphenoidal bone)   ►

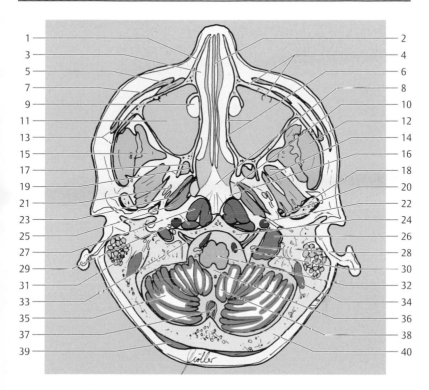

9 Nasolacrimal duct
10 Pharyngotympanic tube (auditory tube)
11 Maxillary sinus
12 Masseter muscle
13 Zygomatic bone and zygomaticus muscles
14 Lateral pterygoid muscle (superior and inferior heads)
15 Temporal muscles
16 Pharyngeal recess
17 Medial pterygoid muscle
18 Head of mandible
19 Pterygoid process (medial and lateral plates)
20 Sphenoidal bone (tip)
21 Mandibular nerve and auriculotemporal nerve
22 Internal carotid artery
23 Tensor veli palatini muscle
24 Clivus
25 Levator veli palatini muscle
26 Internal jugular vein (bulb)
27 Longus capitis muscle
28 Vagus (X) and accessory (XI) nerves
29 Glossopharyngeal nerve (IX)
30 Vertebral artery
31 Mastoid cells
32 Medulla oblongata
33 Hypoglossal nerve (XII)
34 Sigmoid sinus
35 Hemisphere of cerebellum (posterior lobe)
36 Fourth ventricle (medial aperture)
37 Falx cerebelli with occipital sinus
38 Tonsil of cerebellum
39 Semispinalis capitis muscle
40 Occipital bone

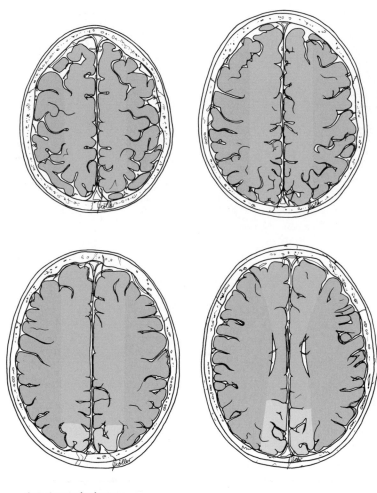

Anterior cerebral artery
Terminal branches

Middle cerebral artery
Terminal branches

Posterior cerebral artery
Terminal branches

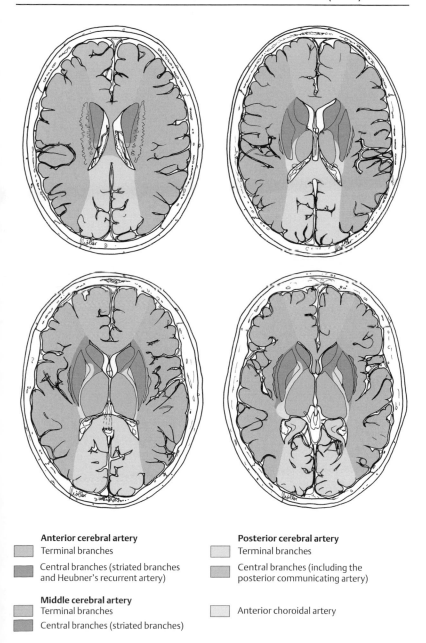

Anterior cerebral artery
Terminal branches

Central branches (striated branches
and Heubner's recurrent artery)

Middle cerebral artery
Terminal branches

Central branches (striated branches)

Posterior cerebral artery
Terminal branches

Central branches (including the
posterior communicating artery)

Anterior choroidal artery

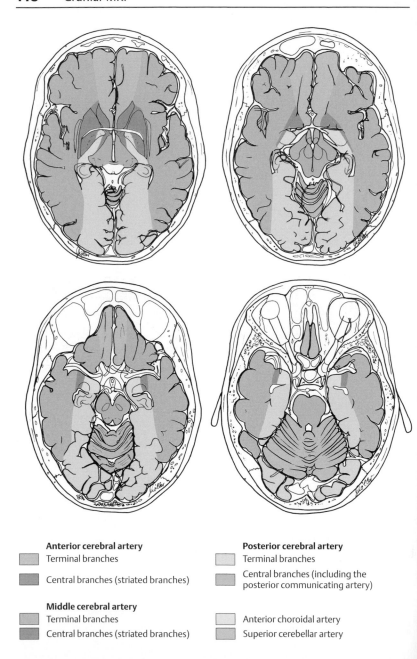

Anterior cerebral artery
Terminal branches

Central branches (striated branches)

Middle cerebral artery
Terminal branches

Central branches (striated branches)

Posterior cerebral artery
Terminal branches

Central branches (including the posterior communicating artery)

Anterior choroidal artery

Superior cerebellar artery

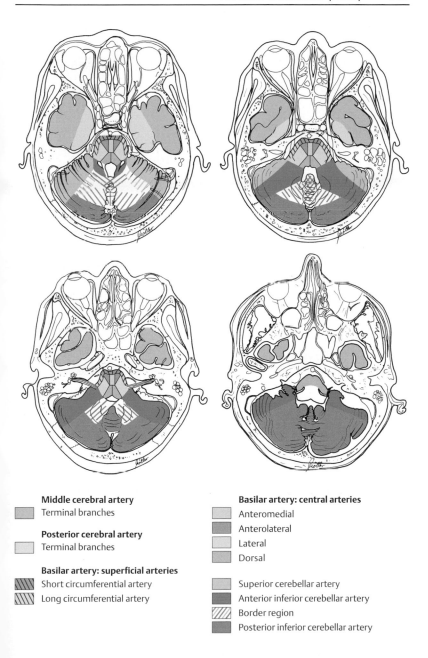

Middle cerebral artery
Terminal branches

Posterior cerebral artery
Terminal branches

Basilar artery: superficial arteries
Short circumferential artery
Long circumferential artery

Basilar artery: central arteries
Anteromedial
Anterolateral
Lateral
Dorsal

Superior cerebellar artery
Anterior inferior cerebellar artery
Border region
Posterior inferior cerebellar artery

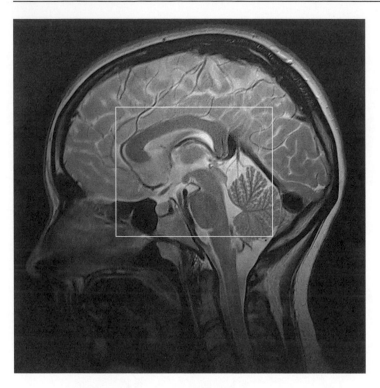

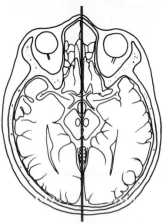

- Frontal lobe
- Parietal lobe
- Occipital lobe
- Cerebellum
- Mesencephalon
- Pons
- Medulla oblongata

1 Superior frontal gyrus
2 Parietal bone and coronal suture
3 Frontal bone
4 Superior sagittal sinus
5 Cingulate gyrus and sulcus
6 Precentral gyrus
7 Corpus callosum (genu)   ▶

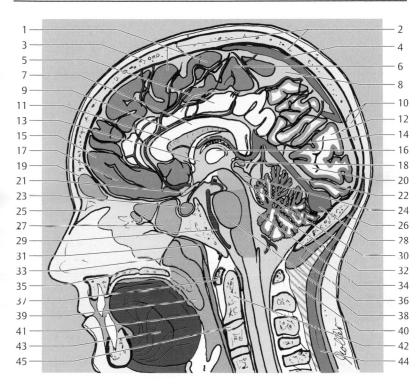

8 Falx cerebri in longitudinal cerebral fissure
9 Pericallosal artery
10 Occipital bone and lambdoid suture
11 Septum pellucidum
12 Cuneus
13 Third ventricle
14 Parieto-occipital sulcus
15 Frontal pole
16 Interthalamic adhesion
17 Straight gyrus
18 Cerebral epiphysis
19 Frontal sinus
20 Lingual gyrus
21 Optic nerve (II)
22 Straight sinus
23 Pituitary gland
24 Quadrigeminal plate
25 Nasal bone
26 External occipital protuberance

27 Ethmoid sinus and sphenoidal sinus
28 Confluence of sinuses
29 Basilar artery
30 Aqueduct
31 Superior constrictor muscle of pharynx
32 Cerebellum
33 Nasopharynx
34 Fourth ventricle
35 Hard palate
36 Rectus capitis posterior minor muscle
37 Atlas, anterior arch
38 Pons
39 Uvula
40 Ligamentum nuchae (nuchal ligament)
41 Oropharynx
42 Dens of axis
43 Tongue
44 Semispinalis capitis muscle
45 Intervertebral disc (C2/C3)

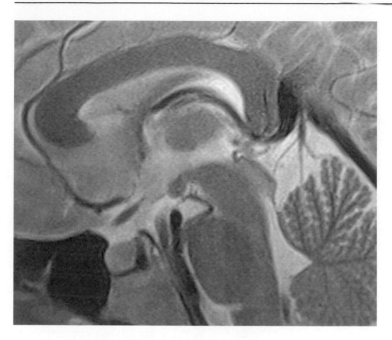

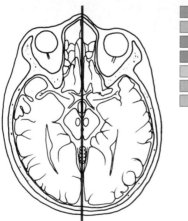

Frontal lobe
Parietal lobe
Occipital lobe
Cerebellum
Mesencephalon
Pons
Medulla oblongata

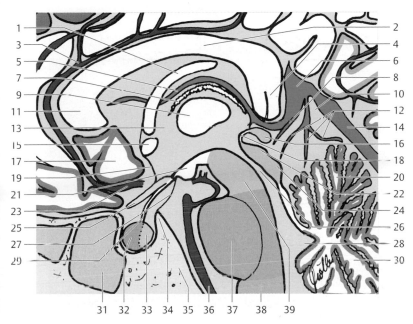

1 Fornix (body)
2 Corpus callosum (trunk)
3 Pericallosal artery
4 Great cerebral vein
5 Internal cerebral vein
6 Corpus callosum (splenium)
7 Choroid plexus
8 Basal vein
9 Interthalamic adhesion
10 Cistern of great cerebral vein
11 Corpus callosum (genu)
12 Cerebellar veins
13 Third ventricle
14 Straight sinus
15 Anterior commissure
16 Pineal body
17 Paraterminal gyrus
18 Posterior commissure
19 Lamina terminalis
20 Hemisphere of cerebellum
   (anterior lobe)
21 Mammillary body

22 Tectal (quadrigeminal) plate (superior
   colliculus)
23 Anterior cerebral artery
24 Tectal (quadrigeminal) plate
   (posterior colliculus)
25 Optic nerve (II)
26 Aqueduct
27 Liliequist membrane
28 Fourth ventricle (roof)
29 Infundibulum of pituitary gland
30 Hemisphere of cerebellum
   (posterior lobe)
31 Sphenoidal sinus
32 Anterior lobe of pituitary gland
   (adenohypophysis)
33 Posterior lobe of pituitary gland
   (neurohypophysis)
34 Dorsum sellae
35 Clivus
36 Basilar artery
37 Pons
38 Medulla oblongata
39 Mesencephalon (midbrain)

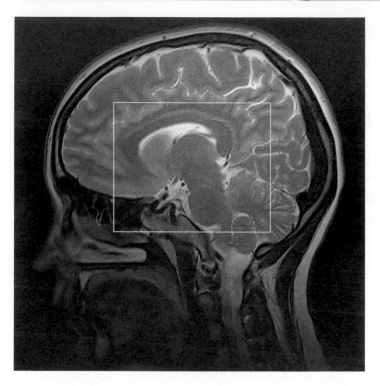

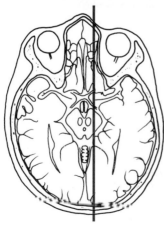

- [ ] Frontal lobe
- [ ] Parietal lobe
- [ ] Occipital lobe
- [ ] Cerebellum
- [ ] Mesencephalon
- [ ] Pons
- [ ] Medulla oblongata

1 Frontal bone and coronal suture
2 Parietal bone
3 Superior frontal gyrus
4 Precentral gyrus
5 Cingulate gyrus
6 Central sulcus
7 Corpus callosum
8 Postcentral gyrus

▶

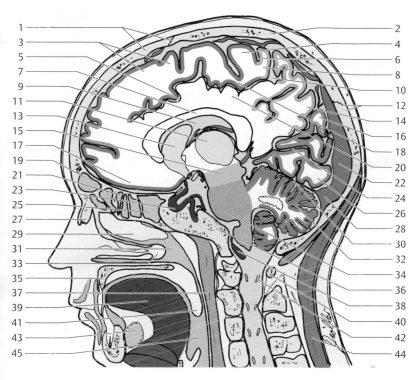

9 Lateral ventricle (central part)
10 Postcentral sulcus
11 Thalamus
12 Occipital bone and lambdoid suture
13 Caudate nucleus (head)
14 Precuneus
15 Cerebral peduncle
16 Cuneus
17 Straight gyrus
18 Precentral lobule
19 Frontal sinus
20 Cingulate gyrus
21 Ethmoidal sinus
22 Superior sagittal sinus
23 Internal carotid artery (siphon)
24 Calcarine sulcus
25 Sphenoidal sinus
26 Medial occipitotemporal gyrus

27 Nasal bone
28 Confluence of sinuses
29 Middle nasal concha
30 Tentorium cerebelli
31 Nasopharynx
32 Cerebellum
33 Inferior nasal concha
34 Pons
35 Hard palate
36 Clivus
37 Longus capitis muscle
38 Vertebral artery
39 Tongue
40 Atlas, posterior arch
41 Uvula
42 Nerve roots
43 Sublingual gland
44 Semispinalis capitis muscle
45 Oropharynx

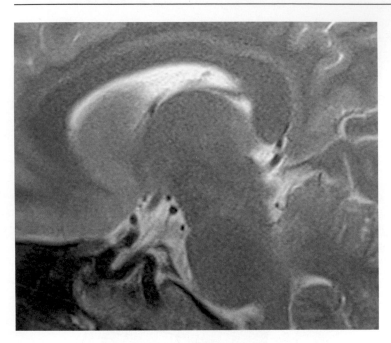

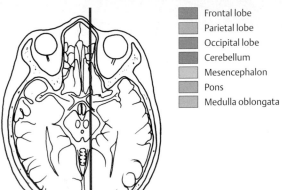

Frontal lobe
Parietal lobe
Occipital lobe
Cerebellum
Mesencephalon
Pons
Medulla oblongata

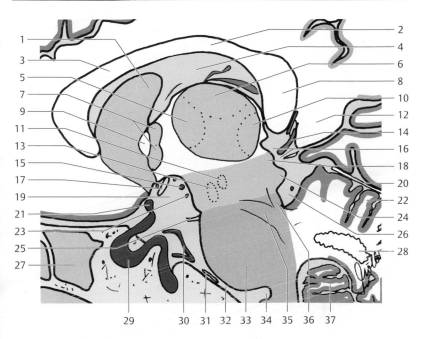

1   Head of caudate nucleus
2   Corpus callosum (trunk)
3   Corpus callosum (genu)
4   Lateral ventricle
5   Thalamus (ventral lateral complex)
6   Thalamus (posterior lateral complex)
7   Globus pallidus (lateral and medial segments)
8   Corpus callosum (splenium)
9   Anterior commissure
10 Thalamus (pulvinar)
11 Red nucleus
12 Parahippocampal gyrus
13 Substantia nigra
14 Great cerebral vein
15 Posterior cerebral artery
16 Quadrigeminal cistern
17 Optic tract
18 Tectal (quadrigeminal) plate (superior colliculus)
19 Interpeduncular cistern
20 Tentorium cerebelli
21 Anterior cerebral artery
22 Hemisphere of cerebellum (anterior lobe)
23 Superior cerebellar artery
24 Tectal (quadrigeminal) plate (posterior colliculus)
25 Trigeminal nerve (V)
26 Ambient cistern
27 Sphenoidal sinus
28 Dentate nucleus
29 Internal carotid artery
30 Posterior communicating artery
31 Abducent nerve (VI)
32 Pontocerebellar cistern
33 Pons
34 Fourth ventricle (lateral aperture)
35 Cerebellar peduncle
36 Lateral lemniscus
37 Tonsil of cerebellum

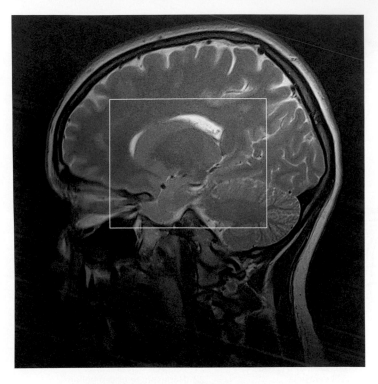

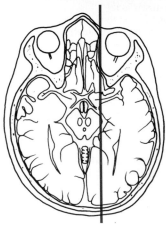

Frontal lobe
Temporal lobe
Parietal lobe
Occipital lobe
Cerebellum
Pons

1 Frontal bone and coronal suture
2 Parietal bone
3 Superior frontal gyrus
4 Precentral gyrus
5 Corpus callosum
6 Postcentral gyrus
7 Caudate nucleus (body)
8 Central sulcus ▶

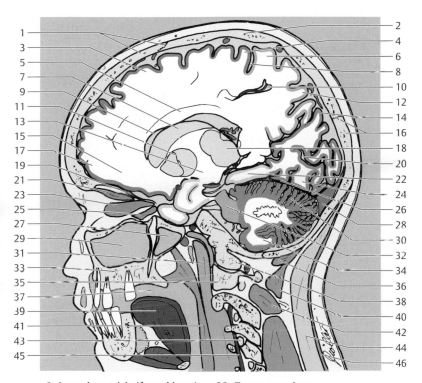

9 Lateral ventricle (frontal horn)
10 Postcentral sulcus
11 Basal nuclei
12 Precuneus
13 Cerebral peduncle
14 Cuneus
15 Orbital gyrus
16 Occipital bone and lambdoid
      suture
17 Inferior frontal gyrus
18 Thalamus
19 Roof of orbit
20 Calcarine sulcus
21 Superior rectus muscle
22 Parahippocampal gyrus
23 Medial rectus muscle
24 Medial occipitotemporal gyrus
25 Inferior rectus muscle
26 Tentorium cerebelli
27 Sphenoidal sinus

28 Transverse sinus
29 Maxillary sinus
30 Superior cerebellar lobe
31 Longus capitis muscle
32 Middle cerebral peduncle
33 Maxilla
34 Inferior cerebellar lobe
35 Atlas, lateral mass
36 Rectus capitis posterior minor muscle
37 Oropharynx
38 Occipital condyle
39 Tongue
40 Rectus capitis posterior major muscle
41 Middle constrictor muscle of pharynx
42 Obliquus capitis inferior muscle
43 Spinal nerve root C4
44 Splenius capitis muscle
45 Vertebral artery
46 Trapezius muscle

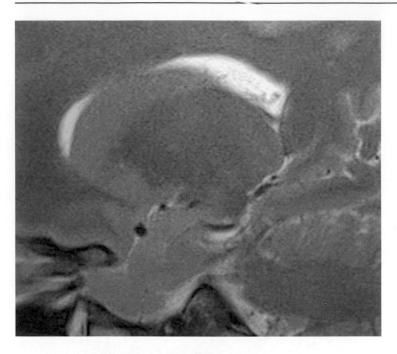

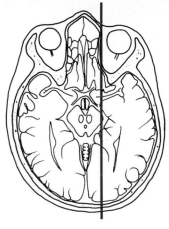

Frontal lobe
Temporal lobe
Parietal lobe
Occipital lobe
Cerebellum
Pons

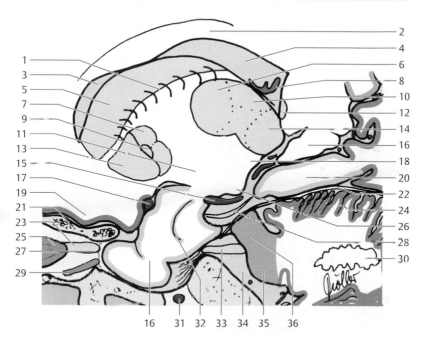

1   Corpus striatum
2   Corpus callosum (trunk)
3   Lateral ventricle (frontal horn)
4   Lateral ventricle
5   Caudate nucleus (head)
6   Thalamus (ventral lateral complex)
7   Globus pallidus
8   Choroid plexus
9   Anterior commissure
10 Thalamus (posterior lateral complex)
11 Internal capsule
12 Fornix (crus)
13 Putamen
14 Thalamus (pulvinar)
15 Posterior cerebral artery
16 Parahippocampal gyrus
17 Middle cerebral artery
18 Medial geniculate body
19 Orbital gyrus
20 Lingual gyrus
21 Sphenoidal bone (lesser wing)
22 Tentorium cerebelli
23 Optic nerve (II)
24 Hemisphere of cerebellum (anterior lobe)
25 Medial rectus muscle
26 Lateral geniculate body
27 Superior orbital fissure
28 Trochlear nerve (IV)
29 Oculomotor nerve (III)
30 Dentate nucleus
31 Internal carotid artery
32 Lateral ventricle (temporal horn)
33 Trigeminal nerve (V)
34 Pontocerebellar cistern
35 Pons
36 Middle cerebellar peduncle

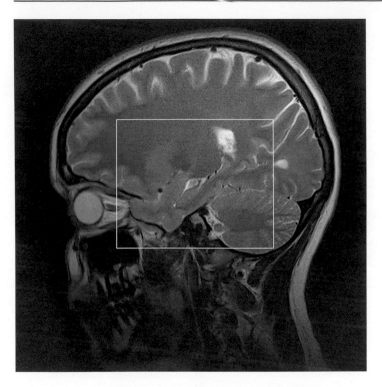

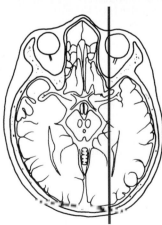

Frontal lobe
Temporal lobe
Parietal lobe
Occipital lobe
Cerebellum

1 Frontal bone and coronal suture
2 Parietal bone
3 Superior frontal gyrus
4 Postcentral gyrus
5 Caudate nucleus (body)
6 Precentral gyrus
7 Thalamus
8 Central sulcus ▶

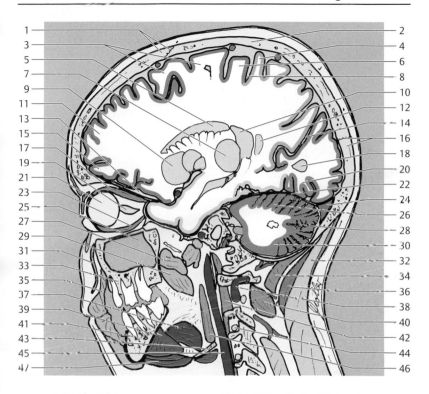

9 Basal nuclei
10 Lateral ventricle
11 Middle frontal gyrus
12 Corpus callosum (major forceps)
13 Roof of orbit
14 Parieto-occipital sulcus
15 Orbital gyrus
16 Occipital bone and lambdoid suture
17 Superior rectus muscle
18 Lateral ventricle (occipital horn)
19 Optic nerve (II)
20 Medial occipitotemporal gyrus
21 Eyeball
22 Tentorium cerebelli
23 Inferior rectus muscle
24 Transverse sinus
25 Maxillary sinus
26 Anterior lobe of cerebellum

27 Levator veli palatini muscle
28 Horizontal fissure
29 Medial pterygoid muscle
30 Posterior lobe of cerebellum
31 Levator labii superioris muscle
32 Splenius capitis muscle
33 Maxilla
34 Rectus capitis posterior major muscle
35 Orbicularis oris muscle
36 Semispinalis capitis muscle
37 Hyoglossus muscle
38 Vertebral artery
39 Mylohyoid muscle
40 Obliquus capitis inferior muscle
41 Mandible
42 Longus capitis muscle
43 Hyoid bone
44 Spinal nerve root C3
45 Internal carotid artery
46 Middle constrictor muscle of pharynx
47 Digastric muscle

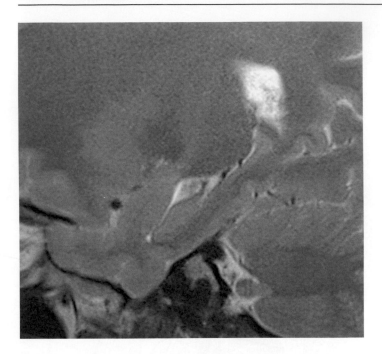

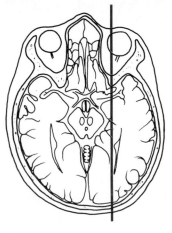

Frontal lobe
Temporal lobe
Parietal lobe
Occipital lobe
Cerebellum

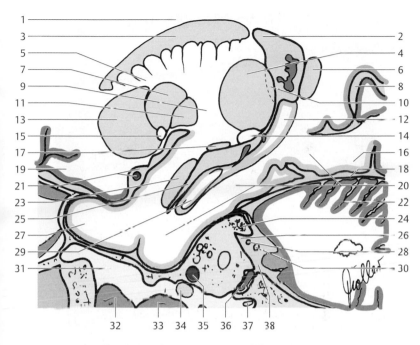

1 Corpus callosum (trunk)
2 Lateral ventricle (central part)
3 Caudate nucleus (body)
4 Thalamus (pulvinar)
5 Internal capsule (anterior limb)
6 Corpus callosum (major forceps)
7 Globus pallidus (lateral segment)
8 Parieto-occipital sulcus
9 Internal capsule (posterior limb)
10 Fornix (crus)
11 Globus pallidus (medial segment)
12 Lateral geniculate body
13 Putamen
14 Subiculum of hippocampus
15 Anterior commissure
16 Medial occipitotemporal gyrus
17 Optic tract
18 Tentorium cerebelli
19 Orbital gyrus
20 Parahippocampal gyrus

21 Middle cerebral artery in cistern of lateral cerebral fossa
22 Hemisphere of cerebellum (anterior lobe)
23 Amygdaloid nucleus
24 Petrous pyramid
25 Lateral ventricle (temporal horn)
26 Internal acoustic meatus
27 Temporal pole
28 Facial nerve (VII)
29 Dentate gyrus
30 Vestibulocochlear (acoustic) nerve (VIII)
31 Infratemporal fossa
32 Medial pterygoid muscle
33 Elevator muscle of the soft palate
34 Pharyngotympanic tube (auditory tube)
35 Internal carotid artery (petrous part)
36 Internal jugular vein in the jugular foramen
37 Hypoglossal nerve (XII) in hypoglossal canal
38 Pontocerebellar cistern

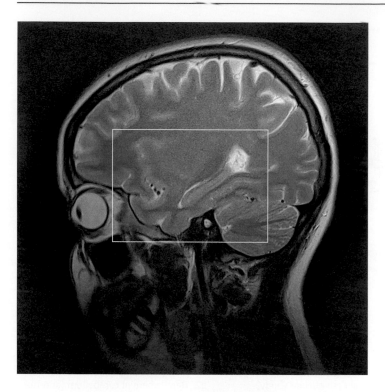

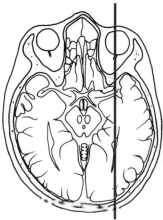

■ Frontal lobe
□ Temporal lobe
■ Parietal lobe
■ Occipital lobe
■ Cerebellum

1 Frontal bone and coronal suture
2 Parietal bone
3 Cerebral white matter (semioval center)
4 Precentral gyrus
5 Superior frontal gyrus
6 Postcentral gyrus
7 Basal ganglia

▶

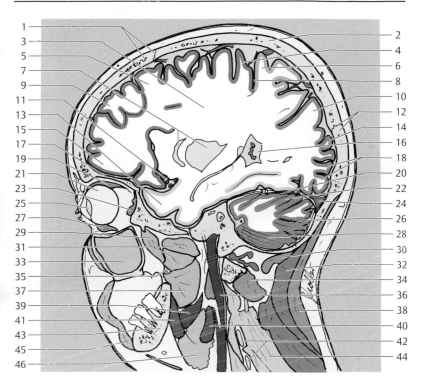

8 Central sulcus
9 Middle frontal gyrus
10 Precuneus
11 Insular arteries
12 Occipital bone and lambdoid suture
13 Temporal pole
14 Cuneus
15 Orbital gyrus
16 Lateral ventricle (occipital horn)
17 Roof of orbit
18 Occipital gyri
19 Superior rectus muscle
20 Tentorium cerebelli
21 Eyeball
22 Anterior lobe of cerebellum
23 Lateral rectus muscle
24 Transverse sinus
25 Lens
26 Horizontal fissure

27 Inferior rectus muscle
28 Posterior lobe of cerebellum
29 Temporal muscle
30 Rectus capitis posterior major muscle
31 Lateral pterygoid muscle
32 Semispinalis capitis muscle
33 Maxillary sinus
34 Obliquus capitis inferior muscle
35 Pterygoid process, lateral plate
36 Internal carotid artery
37 Medial pterygoid muscle
38 Trapezius muscle
39 Styloglossus muscle
40 Digastric muscle
41 Mylohyoid muscle
42 Spinal nerve roots (cervical plexus)
43 Mandible
44 Levator scapulae muscle
45 Orbicularis oris muscle
46 Submandibular gland

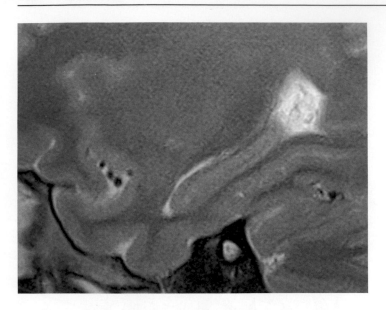

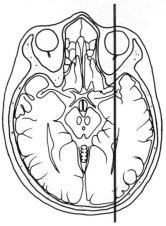

Frontal lobe
Temporal lobe
Cerebellum

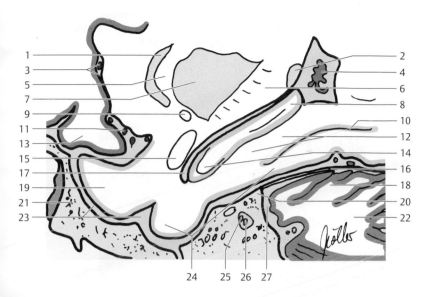

1 Claustrum
2 Caudate nucleus (tail)
3 Insular arteries
4 Lateral ventricle (central part)
   with choroid plexus
5 External capsule
6 Internal capsule
7 Putamen
8 Subiculum of hippocampus
9 Anterior commissure
10 Collateral sulcus
11 Middle cerebral artery
12 Parahippocampal gyrus
13 Orbital gyrus
14 Dentate gyrus
15 Amygdaloid nucleus

16 Tentorium cerebelli
17 Lateral ventricle (temporal horn)
18 Anterior lobe of cerebellum
19 Temporal lobe (temporal pole)
20 Petrous part of temporal bone
   (superior margin)
21 Sphenoidal bone (greater wing)
22 Cerebellum (cerebellar white matter)
23 Middle cranial fossa
24 Medial occipitotemporal gyrus
25 Facial nerve (VII) in internal auditory
   meatus
26 Vestibulocochlear (acoustic) nerve
   (VIII) in internal auditory meatus
27 Pontocerebellar cistern

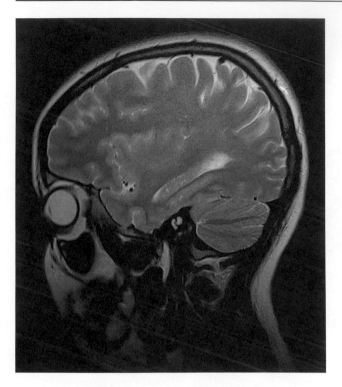

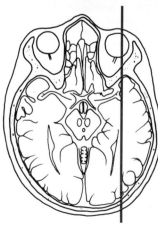

	Frontal lobe
	Temporal lobe
	Parietal lobe
	Occipital lobe
	Cerebellum

1 Frontal bone and coronal suture
2 Parietal bone
3 Middle frontal gyrus
4 Precentral gyrus
5 Inferior frontal sulcus
6 Postcentral gyrus
7 Insular gyri
8 Central sulcus
9 Inferior frontal gyrus
10 Frontal operculum
11 Cistern of lateral cerebral fossa
   (insular cistern) and insular arteries
12 Precuneus ▶

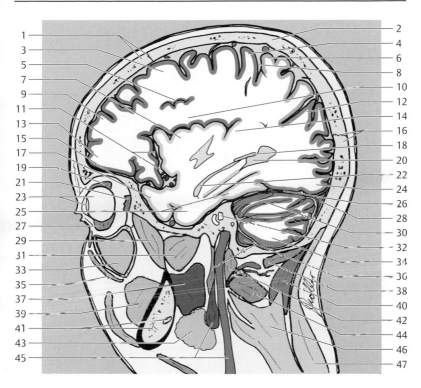

13 Orbital gyrus
14 Transverse temporal gyrus
15 Roof of orbit
16 Occipital bone and lambdoid suture
17 Temporal pole
18 Caudate nucleus (tail)
19 Levator palpebrae superioris muscle
20 Lateral ventricle (occipital horn)
21 Lateral rectus muscle
22 Lateral ventricle (temporal horn)
23 Eyeball and lens
24 Occipital gyri
25 Medial occipitotemporal gyrus
26 Tentorium cerebelli
27 Inferior oblique muscle
28 Transverse sinus
29 Temporal muscle
30 Anterior lobe of cerebellum
31 Lateral pterygoid muscle
32 Internal acoustic meatus
33 Maxillary sinus
34 Posterior lobe of cerebellum
35 Orbicularis oculi muscle
36 Sigmoid sinus and stylopharyngeus muscle
37 Medial pterygoid muscle
38 Rectus capitis posterior major muscle
39 Buccinator muscle
40 Semispinalis capitis muscle
41 Mandible and mandibular canal (inferior alveolar nerve)
42 Atlas (transverse process) and rectus capitis lateralis muscle
43 Submandibular gland
44 Obliquus capitis inferior muscle
45 Internal jugular vein and digastric muscle
46 Levator scapulae muscle
47 Splenius capitis muscle

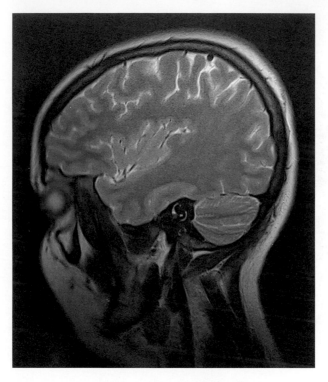

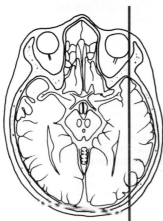

Frontal lobe
Temporal lobe
Parietal lobe
Occipital lobe
Cerebellum

1 Frontal bone and coronal
  suture
2 Parietal bone
3 Middle frontal gyrus
4 Precentral gyrus
5 Inferior frontal sulcus
6 Postcentral gyrus and
  postcentral sulcus
7 Insular gyri
8 Central sulcus

▶

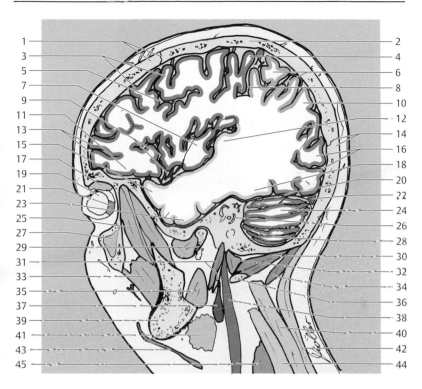

9 Cistern of lateral cerebral fossa (insular cistern) and insular arteries
10 Angular gyrus
11 Orbital gyrus
12 Transverse temporal gyrus
13 Inferior frontal gyrus
14 Occipital bone and lambdoid suture
15 Superior temporal gyrus
16 Occipital gyri
17 Lacrimal gland
18 Inferior temporal gyrus
19 Eyeball
20 Tentorium cerebelli
21 Lateral rectus muscle
22 Transverse sinus
23 Temporal pole and middle temporal gyrus
24 Anterior lobe of cerebellum
25 Temporal muscle

26 Posterior semicircular canal
27 Maxillary sinus
28 Posterior lobe of cerebellum
29 Lateral pterygoid muscle and head of mandible
30 Obliquus capitis superior muscle
31 Styloid muscle and styloid process
32 Rectus capitis lateralis muscle
33 Buccinator muscle
34 Semispinalis capitis muscle
35 Medial pterygoid muscle
36 Atlas, transverse process
37 Digastric muscle, posterior belly
38 Internal jugular vein
39 Mandible
40 Levator scapulae muscle
41 Submandibular gland
42 Splenius capitis muscle
43 Platysma
44 Splenius cervicis muscle
45 Scalenus posterior muscle

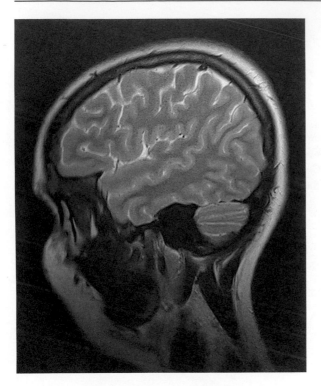

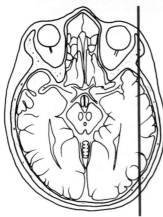

■ Frontal lobe
□ Temporal lobe
■ Parietal lobe
■ Cerebellum

1 Frontal bone and coronal suture
2 Parietal bone
3 Middle frontal gyrus
4 Precentral gyrus
5 Inferior frontal sulcus
6 Postcentral gyrus and
  postcentral sulcus

▶

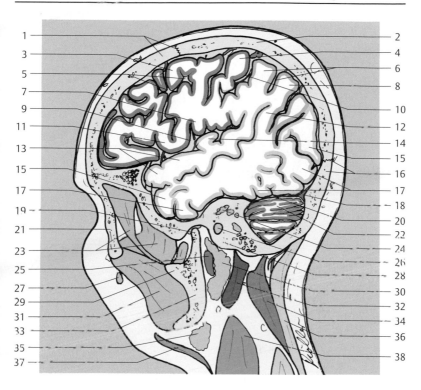

7 Inferior frontal gyrus, insular cortex
8 Supramarginal gyrus
9 Lateral sulcus
10 Central sulcus
11 Inferior frontal gyrus, opercular part
12 Angular gyrus
13 Superior temporal gyrus
14 Transverse temporal gyrus
15 Middle temporal gyrus
16 Occipital bone and lambdoid suture
17 Inferior temporal gyrus
18 Transverse sinus
19 Head of mandible
20 Tentorium cerebelli
21 Zygomatic bone
22 Posterior lobe of cerebellum
23 Temporal muscle
24 Mastoid antrum
25 Retromandibular vein
26 External acoustic meatus
27 Zygomatic muscle
28 Mastoid process
29 Coronoid process
30 Parotid gland
31 Masseter muscle
32 Digastric muscle, posterior belly
33 Mandible (ramus)
34 Semispinalis capitis muscle
35 Submandibular gland
36 Splenius capitis muscle
37 Platysma
38 Sternocleidomastoid muscle

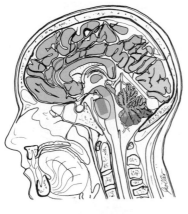
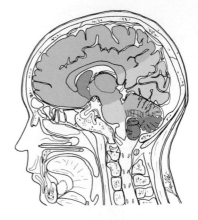
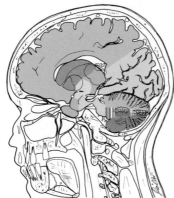
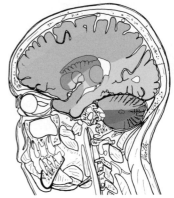

Anterior cerebral artery

Terminal branches

Central branches (striate arteries including distal medial striate artery)

Middle cerebral artery

Terminal branches

Central branches (striate branches)

Posterior cerebral artery

Terminal branches

Central branches (including the posterior communicating artery)

Basilar artery

Anteromedial and anterolateral paramedian branches

Circumferential arteries and lateral and dorsal paramedian branches

Superior cerebellar artery

Anterior superior cerebellar artery

Boundary region

Posterior inferior cerebellar artery

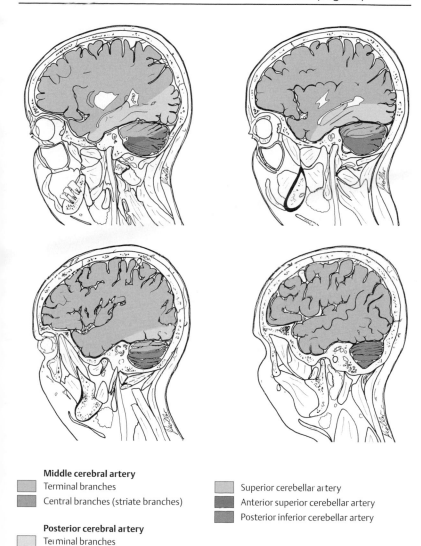

Middle cerebral artery
Terminal branches
Central branches (striate branches)

Posterior cerebral artery
Terminal branches

Anterior choroidal artery

Superior cerebellar artery
Anterior superior cerebellar artery
Posterior inferior cerebellar artery

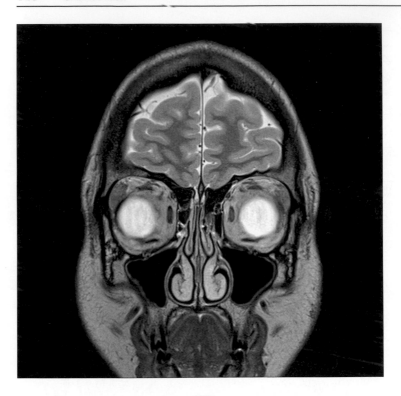

Frontal lobe

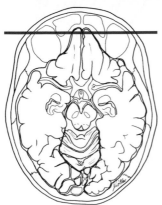

1 Frontal bone
2 Superior sagittal sinus
3 Superior frontal gyrus
4 Falx cerebri
5 Straight gyrus
6 Roof of orbit
7 Middle frontal gyrus

▶

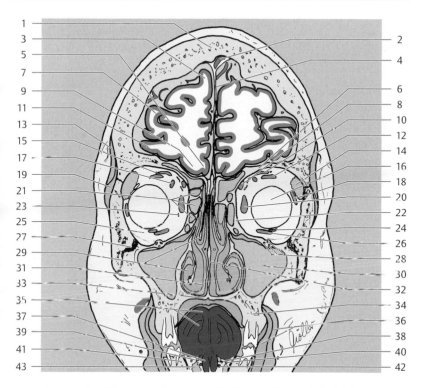

8 Superior oblique muscle
9 Orbital gyri
10 Levator palpebrae superioris muscle
11 Inferior frontal gyrus
12 Superior rectus muscle
13 Temporalis muscle
14 Lacrimal gland
15 Supraorbital nerve (branch of ophthalmic nerve, V_1)
16 Eyeball
17 Superior ophthalmic vein
18 Lateral rectus muscle
19 Orbicularis oculi muscle
20 Medial rectus muscle
21 Ethmoidal cells
22 Orbital plate of ethmoid
23 Ophthalmic artery
24 Inferior rectus muscle
25 Orbit (periorbital fat)
26 Inferior oblique muscle

27 Zygomatic muscle (origin)
28 Infraorbital artery, vein, and nerve (branch of maxillary nerve, V_2)
29 Middle and inferior nasal conchae
30 Maxillary sinus
31 Nasal cavity
32 Nasal septum
33 Hard palate
34 Maxilla (alveolar process)
35 Tongue with intrinsic muscles (longitudinal, transverse, and vertical muscles)
36 Buccinator muscle and buccal mucosa
37 Genioglossus muscle
38 Glossopharyngeal nerve (IX)
39 Sublingual space
40 Submandibular duct
41 Body of mandible
42 Lingual artery
43 Sublingual gland

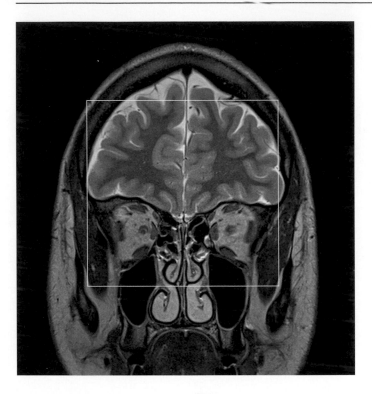

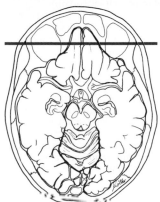

Frontal lobe

1 Frontal bone
2 Superior sagittal sinus
3 Superior frontal gyrus
4 Falx cerebri
5 Cingulate gyrus
6 Interhemispheric fissure
7 Middle frontal gyrus
8 Superior oblique muscle
9 Straight gyrus

▶

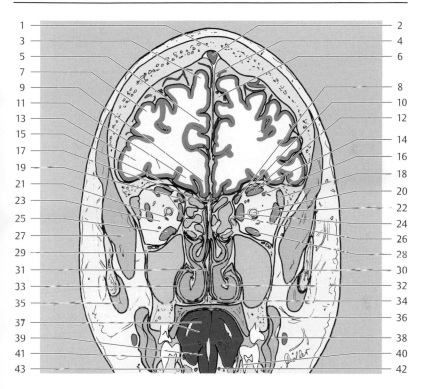

10 Levator palpebrae superioris
    muscle
11 Orbital gyri
12 Superior rectus muscle
13 Inferior frontal gyrus
14 Supraorbital nerve (largest branch
    of frontal nerve, which arises from
    the ophthalmic nerve, V_1)
15 Roof of orbit
16 Superior ophthalmic vein
17 Olfactory bulb
18 Lacrimal gland
19 Ethmoidal cells
20 Optic nerve (II)
21 Ophthalmic artery
22 Lateral rectus muscle
23 Orbit (retrobulbar fat)
24 Medial rectus muscle
25 Infraorbital artery, vein, and nerve
    (branch of maxillary nerve, V_2)

26 Orbital plate of ethmoid
27 Temporalis muscle
28 Inferior rectus muscle
29 Maxillary sinus
30 Zygomatic bone
31 Nasal septum
32 Inferior nasal concha
33 Nasal cavity
34 Hard palate
35 Masseter muscle
36 Maxilla (alveolar process)
37 Tongue with intrinsic muscles (longitudi-
    nal, transverse, and vertical muscles)
38 Buccinator muscle and buccal mucosa
39 Genioglossus muscle
40 Body of mandible
41 Lingual nerve (branch of mandibular
    nerve, V_3) and hypoglossal nerve (XII)
42 Submandibular duct
43 Submandibular gland

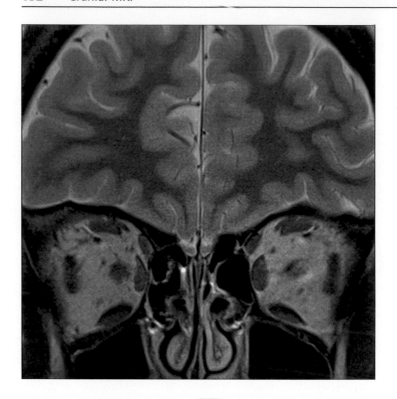

Frontal lobe

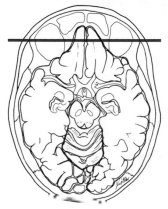

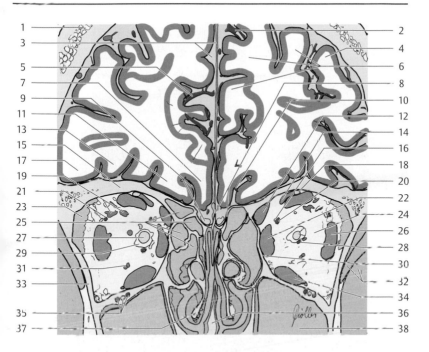

1 Frontal bone
2 Frontal artery (mediomedial branch)
3 Falx cerebri in interhemispheric fissure
4 Middle frontal gyrus
5 Frontal artery (anteromedial branch)
6 Superior frontal gyrus
7 Straight gyrus
8 Crista galli and ethmoidal fovea
9 Olfactory tract (I) and olfactory groove
10 Medial frontobasal artery
11 Medial fronto-orbital gyrus
12 Superior oblique muscle
13 Anterior fronto-orbital gyrus
14 Levator palpebrae superioris muscle
15 Roof of orbit
16 Nasociliary nerve (branch of ophthalmic nerve, V_1)
17 Lateral fronto-orbital gyrus
18 Supraorbital nerve (largest branch of frontal nerve, which arises from the ophthalmic nerve, V_1)
19 Superior ophthalmic vein
20 Ophthalmic artery
21 Lacrimal artery and nerve (branch of ophthalmic nerve, V_1)
22 Medial rectus muscle
23 Lacrimal gland
24 Orbit (retrobulbar fat)
25 Posterior ethmoidal cells
26 Lateral rectus muscle
27 Optic nerve (II)
28 Ophthalmic artery
29 Optic nerve sheath
30 Orbital plate, medial wall of orbit
31 Inferior ophthalmic vein
32 Temporalis muscle
33 Lateral wall of orbit
34 Inferior rectus muscle
35 Infraorbital artery, vein, and nerve (branch of maxillary nerve, V_2)
36 Nasal septum
37 Inferior nasal concha
38 Left maxillary sinus

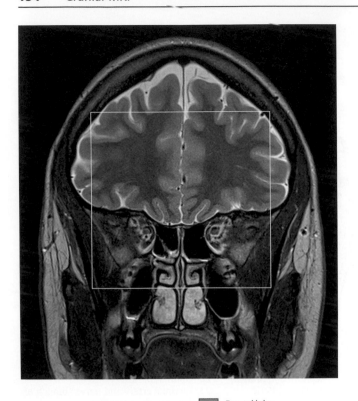

Frontal lobe

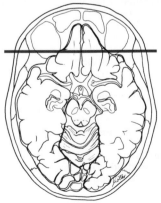

1 Frontal bone
2 Superior sagittal sinus
3 Superior frontal gyrus
4 Falx cerebri in interhemispheric fissure
5 Middle frontal gyrus
6 Callosomarginal artery
7 Cingulate gyrus
8 Straight gyrus

▶

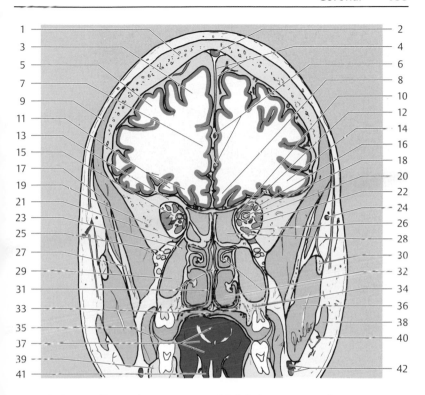

9 Temporalis muscle	26 Inferior rectus muscle
10 Superior oblique muscle	27 Ramus of mandible
11 Orbital gyri	28 Sphenoidal sinus
12 Levator palpebrae superioris and superior rectus muscles	29 Maxillary sinus
13 Roof of orbit	30 Zygomatic arch
14 Inferior frontal gyrus	31 Nasal septum and nasal cavity
15 Orbit	32 Middle and inferior nasal conchae
16 Superior ophthalmic vein	33 Soft palate
17 Temporalis muscle, accessory head	34 Maxilla (alveolar process)
18 Optic nerve (II)	35 Buccinator muscle and buccal mucosa
19 Sphenoid (greater wing)	36 Masseter muscle
20 Medial rectus muscle	37 Tongue with intrinsic muscles (longitudinal, transverse, and vertical muscles)
21 Orbitalis muscle	38 Parotid gland
22 Lateral rectus muscle	39 Body of mandible
23 Pterygopalatine fossa	40 Parotid duct
24 Superficial temporal artery	41 Genioglossus muscle
25 Maxillary nerve (V_2)	42 Facial artery and vein

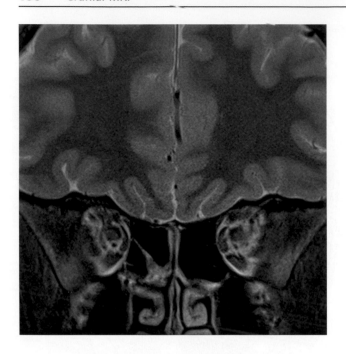

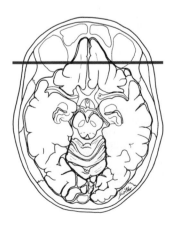

Frontal lobe

1 Cingulate gyrus
2 Falx cerebri in interhemispheric fissure
3 Frontal artery (mediomedial branch)
4 Olfactory tract (I)
5 Cingulate gyrus   ▶

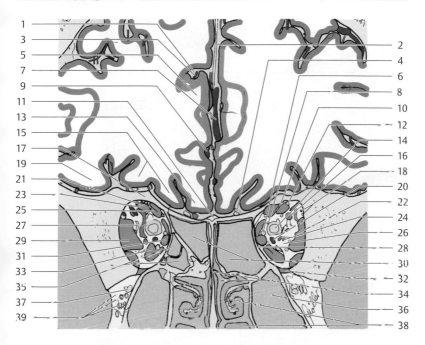

6 Oculomotor nerve, inferior branch (III)
7 Callosomarginal artery
8 Nasociliary nerve (branch of ophthalmic nerve, V₁)
9 Polar frontal artery
10 Trochlear nerve (IV)
11 Sphenoidal crest (crista galli)
12 Frontal nerve (branch of ophthalmic nerve, V₁)
13 Straight gyrus
14 Optic nerve (II)
15 Medial fronto-orbital gyrus
16 Superior ophthalmic vein
17 Roof of orbit
18 Lacrimal artery and nerve (branch of ophthalmic nerve, V₁)
19 Lateral fronto-orbital gyrus
20 Ophthalmic artery
21 Levator palpebrae superioris muscle

22 Abducent nerve (VI)
23 Superior rectus muscle
24 Inferior ophthalmic vein
25 Superior oblique muscle
26 Retro-orbital fat in orbital cone
27 Dural nerve sheath with subarachnoid fluid around optic nerve
28 Orbital plate of ethmoid
29 Lateral rectus muscle
30 Sphenoidal sinus
31 Medial rectus muscle
32 Inferior orbital fissure with orbitalis muscle
33 Inferior rectus muscle
34 Nasal septum and nasal cavity
35 Ethmoidal cells
36 Maxillary sinus
37 Infraorbital nerve (branch of maxillary nerve, V₂)
38 Middle and inferior nasal conchae
39 Pterygopalatine fossa and pterygopalatine ganglion

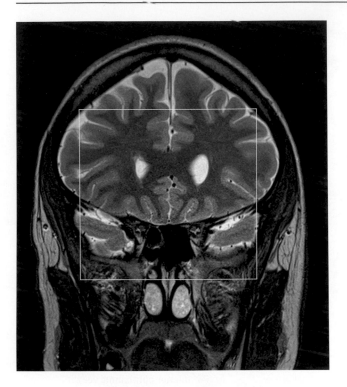

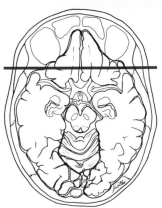

Frontal lobe

Temporal lobe

1 Frontal bone
2 Superior sagittal sinus
3 Superior frontal gyrus
4 Falx cerebri in interhemispheric
  fissure ▶

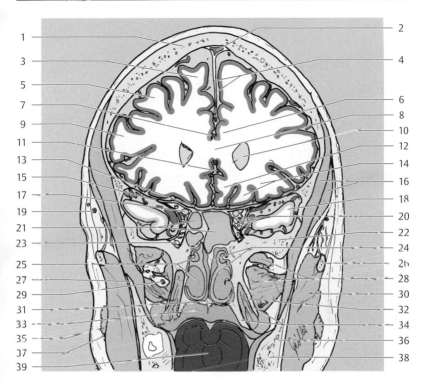

5 Middle frontal gyrus
6 Cingulate gyrus
7 Pericallosal artery
8 Corpus callosum (genu)
9 Inferior frontal gyrus
10 Lateral ventricle (frontal horn)
11 Callosomarginal artery
12 Straight gyrus
13 Olfactory tract
14 Orbital gyri
15 Sphenoid (wing)
16 Temporalis muscle
17 Optic nerve (II)
18 Temporal lobe (pole)
19 Superficial temporal artery
20 Ophthalmic nerve (V₁), oculo-
    motor nerve (III), abducent
    nerve (VI)
21 Ethmoidal cells
22 Temporal bone

23 Maxillary nerve (V₂)
24 Nasal septum and nasal cavity
25 Middle and inferior nasal conchae
26 Zygomatic arch
27 Coronoid process
28 Lateral pterygoid muscle
29 Maxillary artery
30 Masseter muscle
31 Maxilla (hard palate)
32 Medial pterygoid muscle
33 Soft palate
34 Pterygoid process (medial and lateral
    plates)
35 Parotid gland
36 Inferior alveolar artery, vein, and
    nerve (branch of mandibular nerve,
    V₃) in mandibular canal
37 Parotid duct
38 Ramus of mandible
39 Tongue

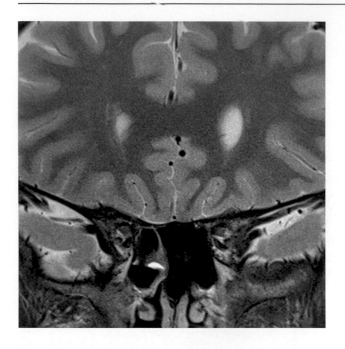

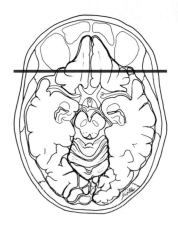

■ Frontal lobe
□ Temporal lobe

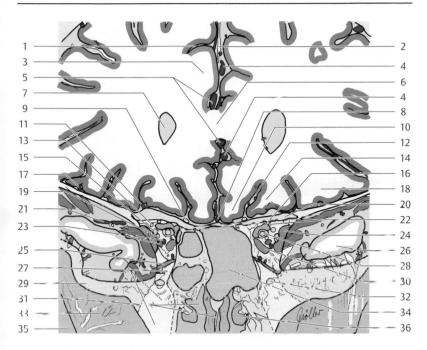

1 Cingulate sulcus
2 Falx cerebri in interhemispheric fissure
3 Cingulate gyrus
4 Callosomarginal artery
5 Pericallosal artery
6 Corpus callosum (genu)
7 Lateral ventricle (frontal horn)
8 Polar frontal artery
9 Olfactory tract
10 Straight gyrus
11 Medial frontobasal artery
12 Olfactory groove
13 Ophthalmic nerve (V₁)
14 Medial frontobasal gyrus
15 Oculomotor nerve (III)
16 Levator palpebrae superioris and superior rectus (tendon insertion) muscles
17 Lateral frontobasal artery
18 Lateral frontobasal gyrus
19 Abducent nerve (VI)
20 Sphenoid (lesser wing)
21 Polar temporal artery and vein
22 Trochlear nerve (IV)
23 Ophthalmic artery and vein
24 Lateral rectus muscle
25 Orbitalis muscle
26 Temporal lobe (pole)
27 Pterygopalatine fossa
28 Optic nerve (II)
29 Temporal bone
30 Medial rectus muscle
31 Nasal septum and nasal cavity
32 Maxillary nerve (second division of trigeminal nerve, V₂)
33 Lateral pterygoid muscle
34 Sphenoidal sinus
35 Temporalis muscle
36 Middle nasal concha

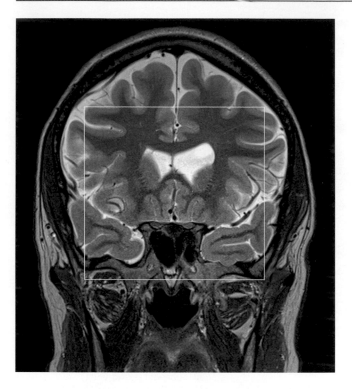

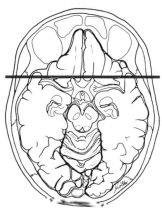

Frontal lobe
Temporal lobe

1 Frontal bone
2 Superior sagittal sinus
3 Superior frontal gyrus
4 Falx cerebri in interhemispheric fissure
5 Middle frontal gyrus
6 Callosomarginal artery ▶

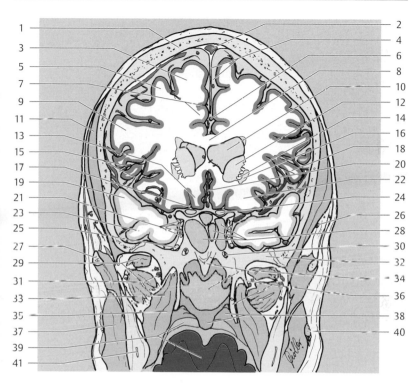

7 Cingulate sulcus and cingulate gyrus
8 Corpus callosum (trunk)
9 Inferior frontal gyrus
10 Lateral ventricle (frontal horn)
11 Temporalis muscle
12 Head of caudate nucleus
13 Straight gyrus
14 Internal capsule (anterior crus)
15 Insular arteries
16 Putamen
17 Olfactory tract (I)
18 Frontal operculum
19 Superior temporal gyrus
20 Anterior cerebral artery
21 Trochlear nerve (IV), oculomotor nerve (III), ophthalmic nerve (V_1), abducent nerve (VI)
22 Orbital gyri
23 Middle temporal gyrus
24 Optic nerve (II)
25 Maxillary nerve (V_2)

26 Superficial temporal artery
27 Zygomatic arch
28 Sphenoidal sinus
29 Lateral pterygoid muscle in infratemporal fossa
30 Pterygoid (vidian) canal
31 Maxillary artery
32 Temporal bone
33 Medial pterygoid muscle
34 Vomer and nasopharynx
35 Tensor veli palatini muscle
36 Pterygoid process (medial and lateral plates)
37 Masseter muscle
38 Uvula and soft palate
39 Tongue and oral cavity
40 Parotid gland and parotid duct
41 Ramus of mandible with inferior alveolar artery, vein, and nerve (branch of mandibular nerve, V_3) in mandibular canal

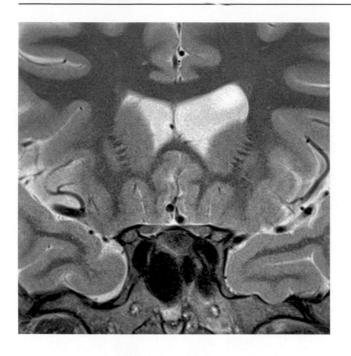

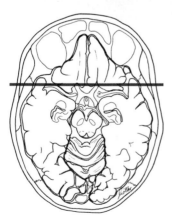

■ Frontal lobe
☐ Temporal lobe

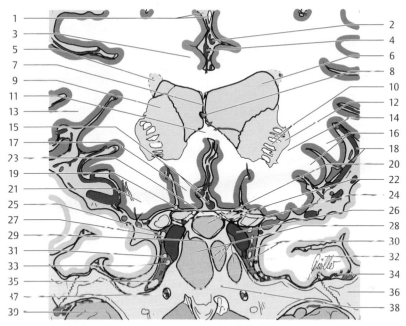

1 Falx cerebri in interhemispheric fissure
2 Callosomarginal artery
3 Cingulate gyrus
4 Pericallosal artery
5 Subependymal layer
6 Lateral ventricle (frontal horn)
7 Septum pellucidum
8 Superior thalamostriate vein
9 Head of caudate nucleus
10 Internal capsule (anterior crus with gray bridges)
11 Corpus callosum (genu)
12 Putamen
13 Inferior frontal gyrus (frontal operculum)
14 External capsule
15 Anterior cerebral artery, A2 segment
16 Insula
17 Straight gyrus
18 Insular arteries
19 Olfactory tract (I)
20 Pituitary gland
21 Orbital gyri (posterior orbitofrontal gyrus)
22 Optic nerve (II) with ophthalmic artery in optic canal
23 Sellar diaphragm
24 Anterior clinoid process
25 Trochlear nerve (IV)
26 Internal carotid artery (siphon)
27 Oculomotor nerve (III)
28 Sphenoidal sinus and septum
29 Floor of sella (sphenoidal bone)
30 Cavernous sinus
31 Ophthalmic nerve (V_1)
32 Middle temporal gyrus
33 Abducent nerve (VI)
34 Middle cerebral artery (temporal branch)
35 Maxillary nerve (V_2)
36 Parietal bone
37 Pterygoid (vidian) canal with artery and vein of pterygoid canal (vidian artery and vein)
38 Sphenoid (body)
39 Lateral pterygoid muscle in infratemporal fossa

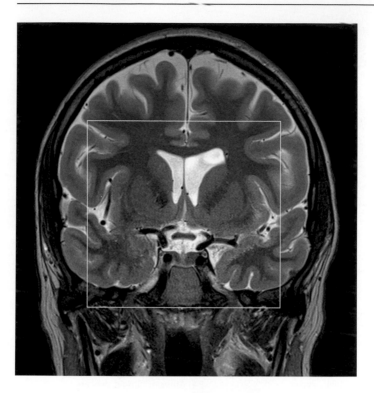

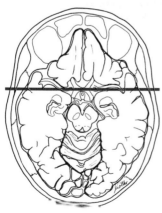

■ Frontal lobe
□ Temporal lobe

1 Frontal bone
2 Superior sagittal sinus
3 Falx cerebri in interhemispheric fissure
4 Superior frontal gyrus
5 Pericallosal artery and callosomarginal artery (anteromedial frontal branch)
6 Cingulate gyrus
7 Corpus callosum (genu)
8 Middle frontal gyrus
9 Lateral ventricle (frontal horn)
10 Septum pellucidum ▶

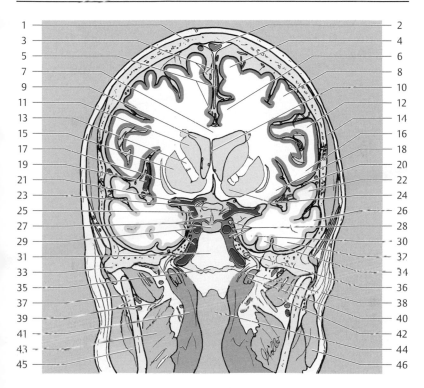

11 Head of caudate nucleus
12 Inferior frontal gyrus
13 Internal capsule (anterior crus)
14 Temporalis muscle
15 Putamen
16 Temporal operculum
17 Claustrum
18 Insula
19 Insular arteries
20 Lateral sulcus
21 Middle cerebral artery
22 Superior temporal gyrus
23 Optic chiasm
24 Nucleus accumbens
25 Internal carotid artery
26 Middle temporal gyrus
27 Pituitary gland with stalk
28 Trochlear nerve (IV), oculomotor
   nerve (III), ophthalmic nerve (V₁),
   abducent nerve (VI)

29 Internal carotid artery (siphon)
30 Parahippocampal gyrus
31 Clivus
32 Inferior temporal gyrus
33 Temporal bone (zygomatic process)
34 Lateral occipitotemporal gyrus
35 Sphenoid (body)
36 Trigeminal ganglion (V) in trigeminal cave
37 Mandible
38 Auditory (eustachian) tube
39 Mandibular artery, vein, and nerve (V₃)
40 Levator veli palatini muscle
41 Pharyngeal constrictor muscle
42 Lateral pterygoid muscle
43 Medial pterygoid muscle
44 Pharynx
45 Masseter muscle
46 Parotid gland

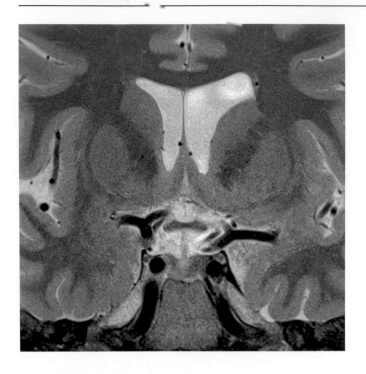

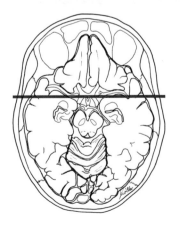

Frontal lobe
Temporal lobe

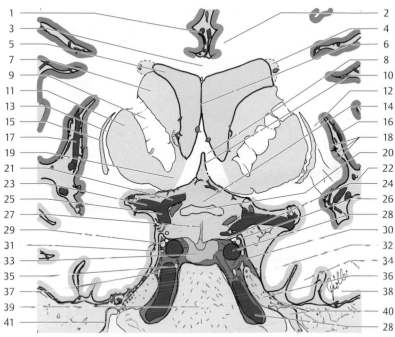

1 Pericallosal artery in interhemispheric fissure
2 Cingulate gyrus
3 Corpus callosum (trunk)
4 Subependymal layer
5 Lateral ventricle (frontal horn)
6 Septum pellucidum
7 Head of caudate nucleus
8 Precommissural fornix
9 Internal capsule (anterior crus)
10 Interhemispheric fissure
(cistern of lamina terminalis)
11 Putamen
12 Extreme capsule
13 External capsule
14 Chiasmatic cistern
15 Claustrum
16 Frontal operculum
17 Insular arteries
18 Insula
19 Nucleus accumbens
20 Optic chiasm
21 Anterior cerebral artery, A1 segment
22 Cistern of lateral cerebral fossa
23 Middle cerebral artery, M1 segment
24 Sellar diaphragm
25 Internal carotid artery
26 Posterior clinoid process
27 Infundibulum
28 Internal carotid artery (siphon)
29 Oculomotor nerve (III)
30 Cavernous sinus
31 Trochlear nerve (IV)
32 Parahippocampal gyrus
33 Pituitary gland
34 Lateral occipitotemporal gyrus
35 Ophthalmic nerve (V₁)
36 Trigeminal cave (Meckel)
37 Abducent nerve (VI)
38 Inferior temporal gyrus
39 Clivus
40 Trigeminal ganglion (V, Gasser) with
fascicles
41 Mandibular nerve (V₃) in foramen
ovale

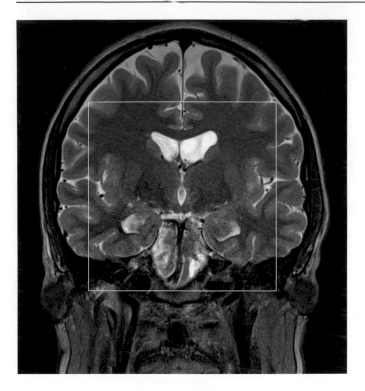

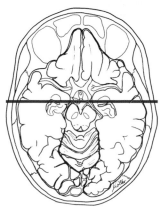

■ Frontal lobe
■ Temporal lobe
■ Pons

1 Parietal bone and sagittal suture
2 Superior sagittal sinus
3 Falx cerebri in interhemispheric
   fissure
4 Superior frontal gyrus
5 Cingulate gyrus
6 Middle frontal gyrus
7 Corpus callosum (trunk)
8 Semioval center
9 Body of caudate nucleus
10 Lateral ventricle (frontal horn)
11 Interventricular foramen (Monro) ▶

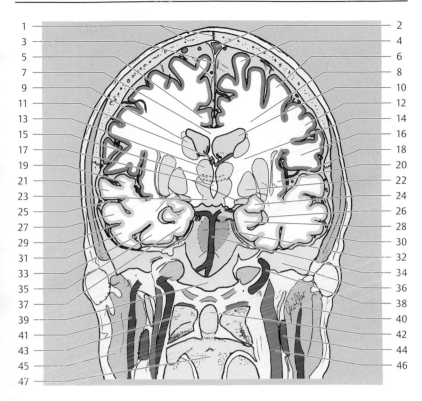

12 Inferior frontal gyrus
13 Thalamus
14 Internal capsule (genu)
15 Anterior commissure
16 Frontal operculum
17 Third ventricle and optic tract
18 Lateral sulcus
19 Transverse temporal gyrus (Heschl)
20 Insula
21 Superior temporal gyrus
22 Basal ganglia (lentiform nucleus)
23 Mammillary body and hypothalamus
24 Amygdala
25 Superior temporal sulcus
26 Lateral ventricle (temporal horn)
27 Middle temporal gyrus

28 Hippocampus
29 Inferior temporal sulcus
30 Temporalis muscle
31 Inferior temporal gyrus
32 Tentorium cerebelli
33 Occipitotemporal sulcus
34 Basilar artery
35 Lateral occipitotemporal gyrus
36 Temporal bone
37 Parahippocampal gyrus
38 Internal carotid artery (siphon)
39 Occipital bone (basilar part), clivus
40 Styloid process
41 External carotid artery
42 Dens of axis
43 Atlas (lateral mass)
44 Digastric muscle (posterior belly)
45 Parotid gland
46 Internal jugular vein
47 Axis

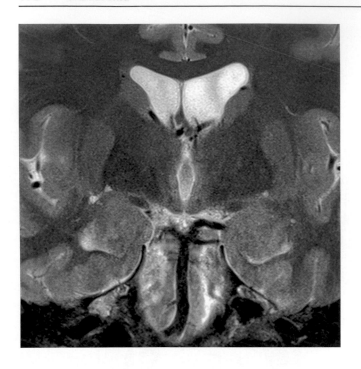

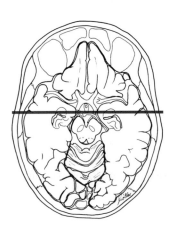

Frontal lobe
Temporal lobe

1 Cingulate gyrus
2 Interhemispheric fissure
3 Subependymal layer
4 Pericallosal artery
5 Lateral ventricle (frontal horn)
6 Corpus callosum (trunk)
7 Body of caudate nucleus
8 Septum pellucidum
9 Superior thalamostriate vein
10 Fornix

▶

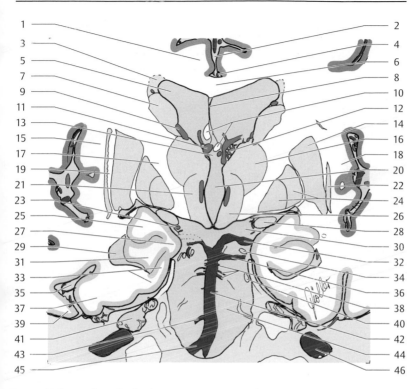

11 Internal cerebral vein
12 Choroid plexus
13 Interventricular foramen (Monro)
14 Putamen
15 Extreme capsule
16 Thalamus (ventral anterior nucleus)
17 Internal capsule (genu)
18 Insula
19 External capsule
20 Third ventricle and fornix (column)
21 Hypothalamus
22 Claustrum
23 Basilar vein
24 Globus pallidus, lateral and medial segments
25 Amygdaloid body
26 Mammillary body
27 Uncus (parahippocampal gyrus)

28 Optic tract
29 Lateral ventricle (temporal horn)
30 Ambient cistern
31 Pes hippocampi
32 Posterior cerebral artery
33 Parahippocampal gyrus
34 Oculomotor nerve (III)
35 Occipitotemporal sulcus
36 Superior cerebellar artery
37 Lateral occipitotemporal gyrus
38 Basilar artery perforators
39 Inferior temporal gyrus
40 Trochlear nerve (IV)
41 Trigeminal nerve (ganglion, V) in trigeminal cave (Meckel)
42 Basilar artery
43 Anterior inferior cerebellar artery (AICA)
44 Pontine cistern
45 Vertebral artery
46 Internal carotid artery (siphon)

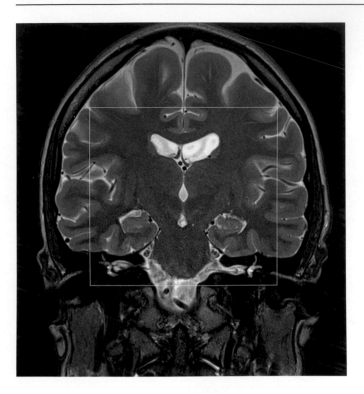

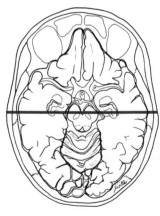

Frontal lobe

Temporal lobe

Parietal lobe

Mesencephalon

Pons

1 Parietal bone
2 Superior sagittal sinus
3 Superior frontal gyrus
4 Falx cerebri
5 Cingulate gyrus
6 Precentral gyrus
7 Semioval center
8 Lateral ventricle
9 Corpus callosum (trunk)
10 Central sulcus
11 Caudate nucleus (body)

▶

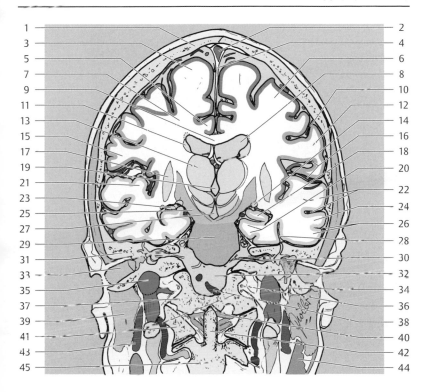

12 Postcentral gyrus
13 Thalamus
14 Optic nerve (II)
15 Parietal operculum
16 Insular arteries in lateral sulcus
17 Basal ganglia (lentiform nucleus)
18 Amygdala
19 Third ventricle
20 Hippocampus and parahippo-campal gyrus
21 Transverse temporal gyrus (Heschl)
22 Superior temporal gyrus and sulcus
23 Lateral ventricle (temporal horn) with choroid plexus
24 Middle temporal gyrus
25 Cerebral peduncle
26 Inferior temporal gyrus and sulcus

27 Interpeduncular cistern
28 Occipitotemporal sulcus
29 Pons
30 Vestibulocochlear nerve (VIII) and facial nerve (VII) in internal acoustic meatus
31 Temporal bone
32 Prepontine cistern
33 External acoustic meatus
34 Facial nerve (VII)
35 Internal jugular vein
36 Hypoglossal nerve (XII)
37 Occipital bone (condyle)
38 Vertebral artery
39 Parotid gland
40 Transverse ligament of atlas
41 Atlas (lateral mass)
42 Dens of axis
43 Digastric muscle (posterior belly)
44 Sternocleidomastoid muscle
45 Axis

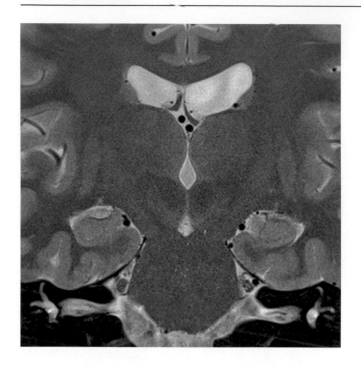

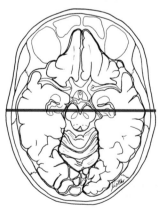

<table>
<tr><td>☐</td><td>Temporal lobe</td></tr>
<tr><td>☐</td><td>Parietal lobe</td></tr>
<tr><td>☐</td><td>Mesencephalon</td></tr>
<tr><td>☐</td><td>Pons</td></tr>
</table>

1 Cingulate gyrus
2 Pericallosal artery
3 Corpus callosum (trunk)
4 Septum pellucidum
5 Fornix (crus)
6 Subependymal layer
7 Caudate nucleus (body)
8 Lateral ventricle
9 Internal cerebral vein ▶

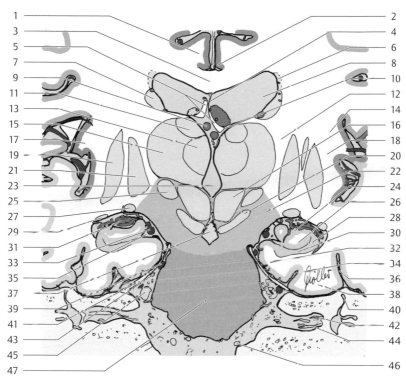

10 Interventricular foramen (Monro)
11 Thalamus (anterior nucleus)
12 Internal capsule (posterior crus)
13 Thalamus (medial nucleus)
14 External capsule
15 Thalamus (ventral lateral nucleus)
16 Red nucleus
17 Insula
18 Extreme capsule
19 Claustrum
20 Substantia nigra
21 Putamen
22 Cerebral peduncle
23 Third ventricle
24 Hippocampus (Ammon's horn)
25 Subthalamic nucleus
26 Dentate gyrus
27 Optic tract (I)
28 Hippocampus (alveus)
29 Caudate nucleus (tail)
30 Subiculum
31 Lateral ventricle (temporal horn)
32 Parahippocampal gyrus
33 Posterior cerebral artery
34 Collateral sulcus
35 Hippocampal sulcus
36 Occipitotemporal sulcus
37 Interpeduncular cistern
38 Lateral occipitotemporal gyrus
39 Superior cerebellar artery
40 Superior semicircular canal
41 Tentorium cerebelli
42 Facial nerve (VII)
43 Trochlear nerve (IV)
44 Vestibulocochlear nerve (VIII) in internal acoustic meatus
45 Trigeminal nerve (V)
46 Abducent nerve (VI)
47 Pons

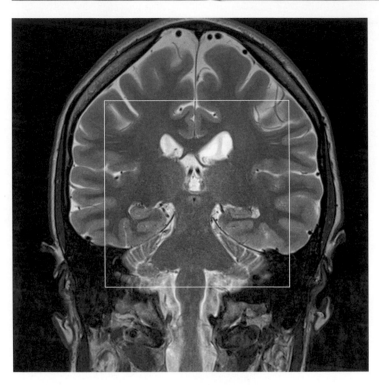

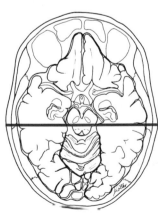

Frontal lobe
Temporal lobe
Parietal lobe
Cerebellum
Mesencephalon
Pons
Medulla oblongata

1 Parietal bone
2 Superior sagittal sinus
3 Superior frontal gyrus
4 Interhemispheric fissure and falx cerebri
5 Paracentral lobe
6 Cingulate gyrus
7 Precentral gyrus

▶

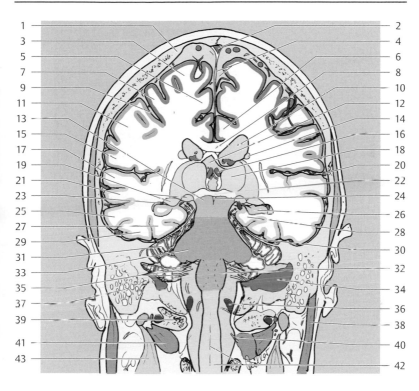

8 Corpus callosum
9 Central sulcus
10 Lateral ventricle
11 Postcentral gyrus
12 Third ventricle
13 Crus cerebri
14 Caudate nucleus
15 Inferior frontal gyrus
16 Internal cerebral vein
17 Transverse temporal gyrus
18 Thalamus
19 Medial and lateral geniculate
 bodies
20 Sylvian fissure
21 Superior temporal gyrus
22 Posterior commissure
23 Lateral ventricle (temporal
 horn)
24 Interpeduncular cistern
25 Medial temporal gyrus

26 Hippocampus
27 Lateral occipitotemporal gyrus
28 Parahippocampal gyrus
29 Inferior temporal gyrus
30 Tentorium cerebelli
31 Anterior lobe of cerebellum
32 Inferior olivary nucleus
33 Middle cerebellar peduncle
34 Sigmoid sinus
35 Facial nerve (VII), vestibulocochlear
 nerve (VIII), glossopharyngeal nerve
 (IX)
36 Vertebral artery and vein
37 Mastoid process with mastoid cells
38 Sternocleidomastoid muscle
39 Atlas (lateral mass)
40 Spinal ganglion (C 2)
41 Obliquus capitis inferior muscle
42 Spinal cord with median fissure
43 Levator scapulae muscle

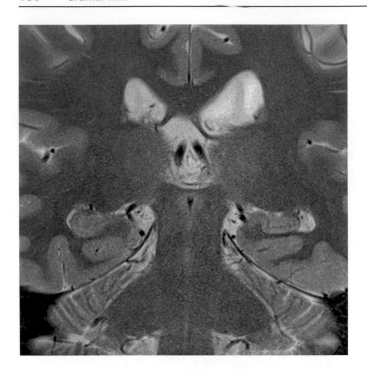

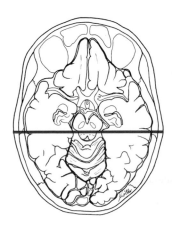

Frontal lobe

Temporal lobe

Parietal lobe

Mesencephalon

Pons

Medulla oblongata

1 Cingulate gyrus
2 Precuneal artery in cingulate sulcus
3 Corpus callosum (trunk)
4 Lateral ventricle
5 Fornix (crus)
6 Third ventricle
7 Caudate nucleus (body)
8 Internal cerebral vein
9 Thalamus (medial nucleus)
10 Suprapineal recess
11 Thalamus (ventral nuclei)
12 Pineal body ▶

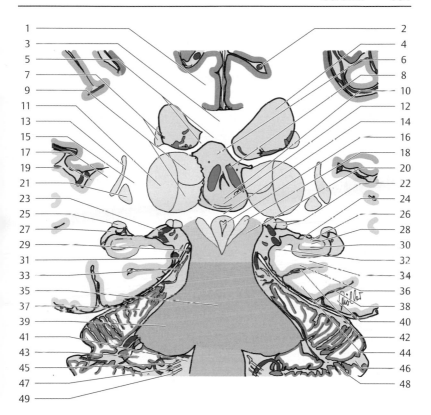

13 Putamen
14 Posterior commissure
15 Internal capsule (posterior crus)
16 Aqueduct of midbrain (aditus)
17 External capsule
18 Substantia nigra
19 Insula
20 Cerebral peduncle
21 Globus pallidus
22 Medial and lateral geniculate
   bodies
23 Posterior cerebral artery in
   ambient cistern
24 Hippocampus (fimbria)
25 Caudate nucleus (tail)
26 Hippocampus (alveus)
27 Lateral ventricle (temporal horn)
28 Hippocampus (Ammon's horn)
29 Superior cerebellar artery
30 Dentate gyrus

31 Tentorium cerebelli
32 Subiculum
33 Trochlear nerve (IV)
34 Collateral white matter
35 Pons
36 Parahippocampal gyrus
37 Anterior lobe of cerebellum
38 Occipitotemporal sulcus
39 Middle cerebellar peduncle
40 Inferior temporal gyrus
41 Pontocerebellar cistern
42 Collateral sulcus
43 Flocculus
44 Lateral occipitotemporal gyrus
45 Facial nerve (VII) with intermediate nerve
46 Horizontal fissure
47 Vestibulocochlear nerve (VIII)
48 Caudal (posterior) lobe of cerebellum
49 Glossopharyngeal nerve (IX) and vagus
   nerve (X)

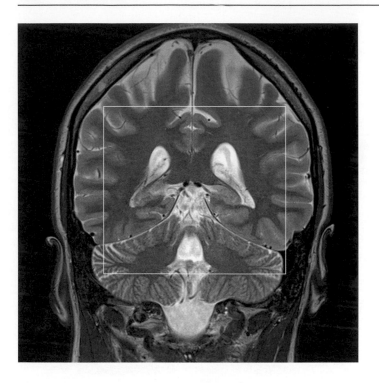

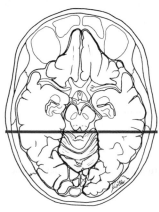

Frontal lobe

Temporal lobe

Parietal lobe

Occipital lobe

Cerebellum

1 Parietal bone
2 Superior sagittal sinus and sagittal suture
3 Superior frontal gyrus
4 Paracentral lobe
5 Interhemispheric fissure and falx cerebri
6 Precentral gyrus
7 Precuneus
8 Central sulcus
9 Corpus callosum
10 Postcentral gyrus
11 Internal cerebral vein
12 Supramarginal gyrus
13 Pineal body (pineal gland) ▶

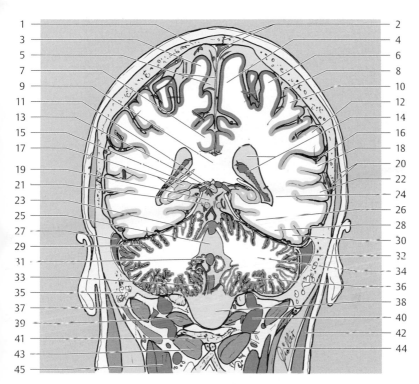

14 Lateral ventricle (trigone) with
   choroid plexus
15 Fornix
16 Lateral sulcus
17 Hippocampus
18 Superior temporal gyrus
19 Quadrigeminal cistern
20 Temporalis muscle and
   squamous suture
21 Superior colliculus of quadrigeminal plate
22 Middle temporal gyrus
23 Cerebellum (anterior lobe,
   quadrangular lobule)
24 Optic radiation
25 Fourth ventricle
26 Medial occipitotemporal gyrus
27 Transverse sinus
28 Lateral occipitotemporal gyrus
29 Posterior superior fissure

30 Inferior temporal gyrus
31 Cerebellar vermis (superior)
32 Cerebellum (posterior lobe, superior
   semilunar lobule)
33 Cerebellar tonsil
34 White matter of cerebellum
35 Temporal bone (mastoid process with
   mastoid cells)
36 Cerebellum (posterior lobe, inferior
   semilunar lobule)
37 Obliquus capitis superior muscle
38 Cerebellomedullary cistern (cisterna
   magna)
39 Rectus capitis posterior major muscle
40 Deep cervical vein
41 Atlas (posterior arch)
42 Sternocleidomastoid muscle
43 Obliquus capitis inferior muscle
44 Splenius capitis muscle
45 Semispinalis capitis muscle

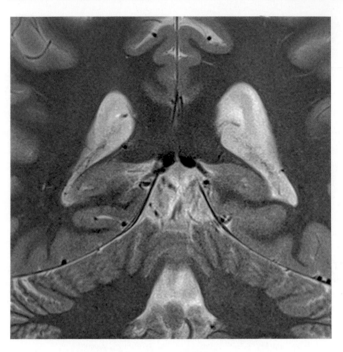

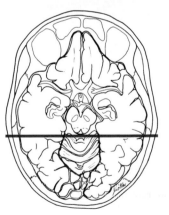

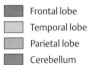

Frontal lobe
Temporal lobe
Parietal lobe
Cerebellum

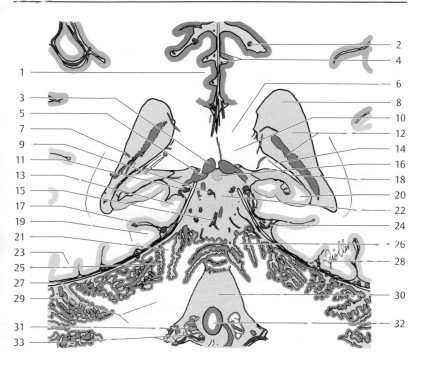

1	Cingulate gyrus
2	Precuneal artery in cingulate sulcus
3	Internal cerebral vein
4	Interhemispheric fissure and falx cerebri
5	Basal vein (Rosenthal)
6	Corpus callosum (splenium)
7	Superior thalamostriate vein
8	Lateral ventricle (trigone)
9	Superior cerebellar artery
10	Commissure (of hippocampus)
11	Medial occipital artery
12	Choroid plexus in lateral ventricle
13	Parahippocampal gyrus
14	Fornix (crus)
15	Superior cerebellar artery
16	Pineal body (pineal gland)
17	Collateral sulcus
18	Hippocampus (fimbria)
19	Lateral occipitotemporal gyrus
20	Hippocampus (tail)
21	Anterior lobe of cerebellum (quadrangular lobule)
22	Cistern of tectal (quadrigeminal) plate
23	Inferior temporal gyrus
24	Lateral occipital artery
25	Primary fissure
26	Vermis of anterior lobe of cerebellum
27	Posterior superior fissure
28	Occipitotemporal sulcus
29	Middle cerebellar peduncle and cerebellar white matter
30	Fourth ventricle
31	Cerebellar tonsil
32	Cerebellar vermis (uvula)
33	Posterior inferior cerebellar artery (PICA)

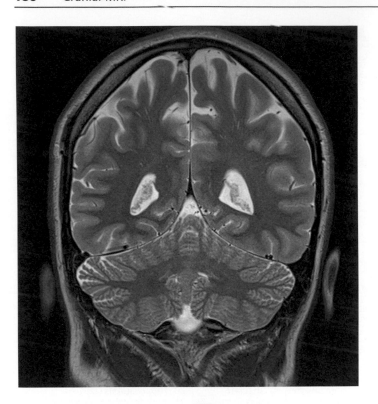

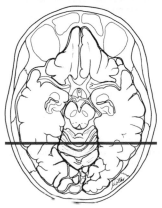

■ Frontal lobe
□ Temporal lobe
□ Parietal lobe
■ Cerebellum

1 Parietal bone and sagittal suture
2 Superior sagittal sinus
3 Precentral gyrus
4 Falx cerebri in interhemispheric fissure
5 Postcentral gyrus
6 Supramarginal gyrus
7 Precuneus
8 Straight sinus
9 Cuneus
10 Superior cerebellar cistern ▶

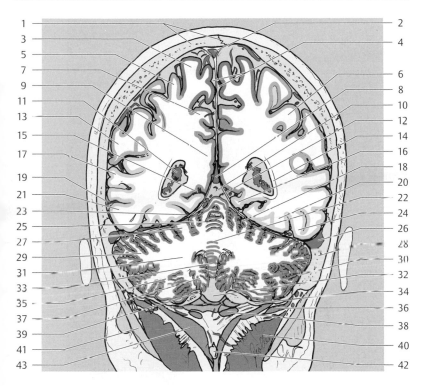

11 Lateral ventricle (occipital horn) with choroid plexus
12 Superior cerebellar artery
13 Frontoparietal operculum
14 Optic radiation
15 Calcarine sulcus
16 Striate area
17 Middle temporal gyrus
18 Incisura prima
19 Superior vermis
20 Medial occipitotemporal gyrus
21 Inferior temporal gyrus
22 Vermis (folium)
23 Tentorium cerebelli
24 Lateral occipitotemporal gyrus
25 Vermis (declive, posterior lobe)
26 Transverse sinus
27 Anterior lobe (quadrangular lobule) of cerebellum
28 Temporal bone

29 Posterior lobe (superior semilunar lobule) of cerebellum
30 Horizontal fissure
31 Cerebellum (white matter with dentate nucleus)
32 Cerebellomedullary cistern (cisterna magna)
33 Inferior vermis (uvula of vermis)
34 Occipital bone
35 Posterior lobe (inferior semilunar lobule) of cerebellum
36 Obliquus capitis superior muscle
37 Cerebellar tonsil
38 Rectus capitis posterior minor muscle
39 Posterior inferior cerebellar artery
40 Semispinalis capitis muscle
41 Splenius capitis muscle
42 Spinous process of axis
43 Rectus capitis posterior major muscle

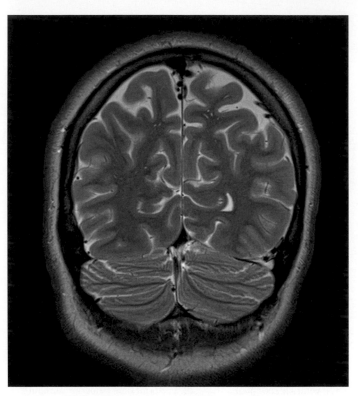

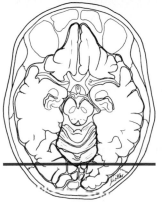

Parietal lobe
Occipital lobe
Cerebellum

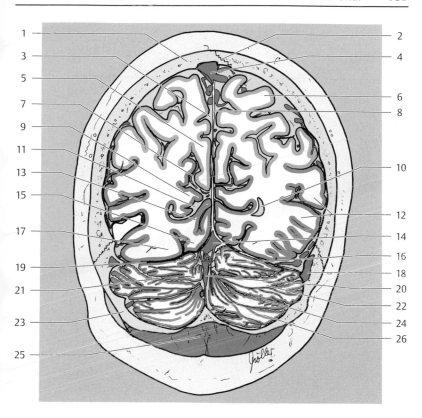

1 Parietal bone
2 Sagittal suture
3 Interhemispheric fissure
4 Superior sagittal sinus
5 Precuneus
6 Angular gyrus
7 Parieto-occipital sulcus
8 Falx cerebri
9 Cuneus
10 Lateral ventricle (occipital horn)
11 Calcarine sulcus
12 Occipital gyri
13 Striate area
14 Straight sinus
15 Medial occipitotemporal gyrus
16 Anterior lobe of cerebellum
17 Lateral occipitotemporal gyrus
18 Transverse sinus
19 Tentorium cerebelli
20 Occipital sinus
21 Posterior superior fissure
22 Posterior lobe of cerebellum (superior semilunar lobule)
23 Occipital bone
24 Horizontal fissure
25 Semispinalis capitis
26 Posterior lobe of cerebellum (inferior semilunar lobule)

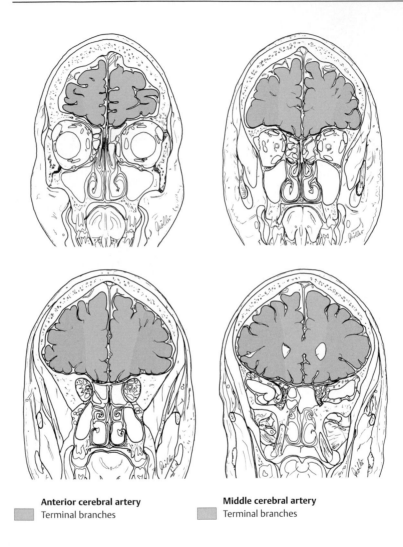

Anterior cerebral artery
Terminal branches

Middle cerebral artery
Terminal branches

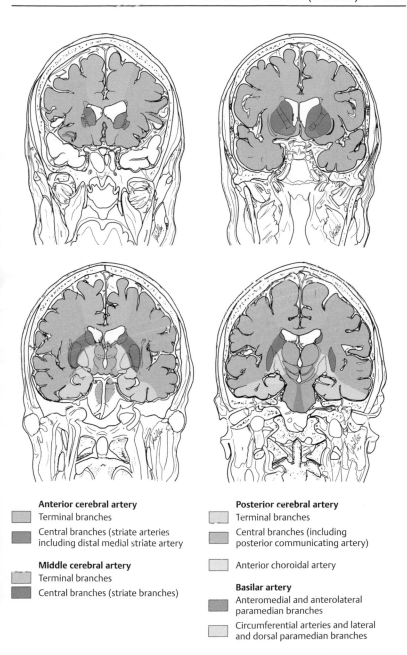

Anterior cerebral artery

Terminal branches

Central branches (striate arteries including distal medial striate artery

Middle cerebral artery

Terminal branches

Central branches (striate branches)

Posterior cerebral artery

Terminal branches

Central branches (including posterior communicating artery)

Anterior choroidal artery

Basilar artery

Anteromedial and anterolateral paramedian branches

Circumferential arteries and lateral and dorsal paramedian branches

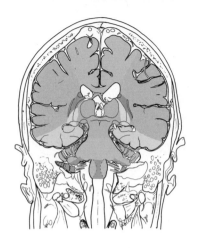
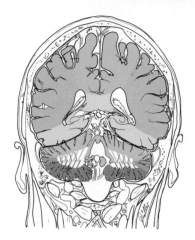
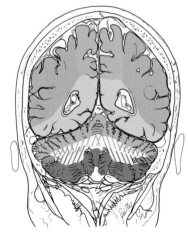
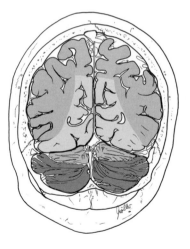

Anterior cerebral artery
Terminal branches

Middle cerebral artery
Terminal branches

Posterior cerebral artery
Terminal branches

Central branches (including posterior communicating artery)

Internal carotid artery
Anterior choroidal artery

Basilar artery
Circumferential arteries and lateral and dorsal paramedian branches

Superior cerebellar artery
Anterior inferior cerebellar artery
Border area
Posterior inferior cerebellar artery

Vertebral artery
Anterior spinal artery

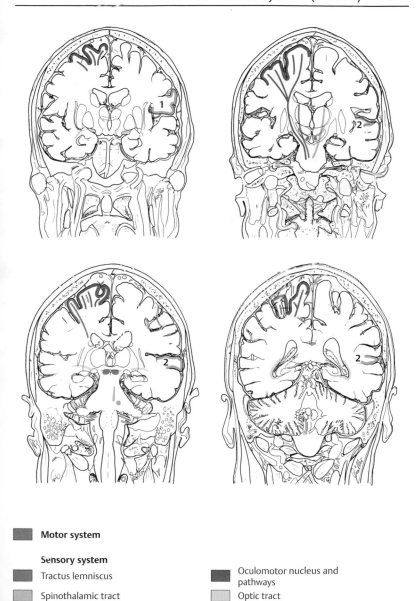

Motor system

Sensory system

Tractus lemniscus

Spinothalamic tract

Mesencephalic nucleus of
trigeminal nerve

Oculomotor nucleus and
pathways

Optic tract

Speech center
(1 = motor, 2 = sensory)

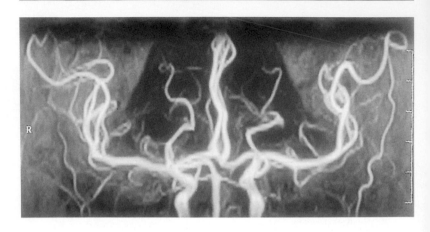

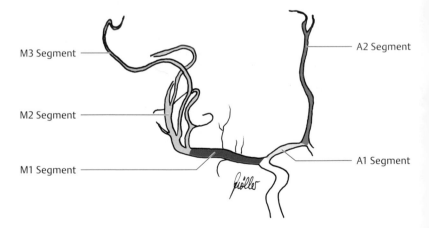

M3 Segment

M2 Segment

M1 Segment

A2 Segment

A1 Segment

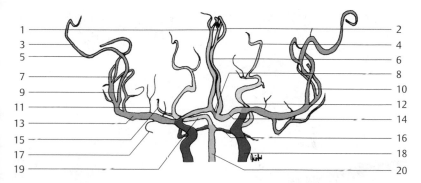

Frontal view

■ Anterior cerebral artery
■ Middle cerebral artery
□ Posterior cerebral artery

1 Callosomarginal artery
2 Pericallosal artery
3 Superior parietal artery
4 Posterior cerebral artery (parieto-occipital ramus)
5 Middle cerebral artery (opercular part, M3 segment)
6 Anterior cerebral artery (postcommunicating part)
7 Insular arteries
8 Anterior communicating artery
9 Middle cerebral artery (insular part, M2 segment)
10 Anterior temporal artery and middle temporal artery

11 Striate artery
12 Left posterior cerebral artery (from internal carotid artery, variant)
13 Middle cerebral artery (sphenoid part, M1 segment)
14 Anterior cerebral artery (precommunicating part)
15 Posterior cerebral artery (temporal and occipitotemporal branches)
16 Superior cerebellar artery
17 Polar temporal artery
18 Internal carotid artery
19 Right posterior cerebral artery
20 Basilar artery

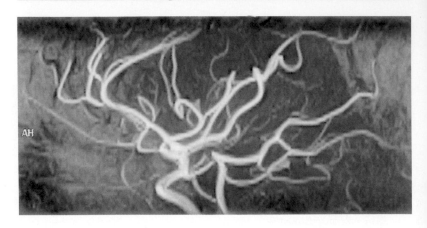

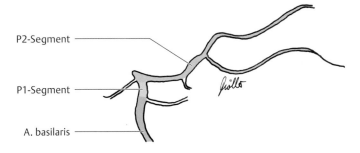

P2-Segment

P1-Segment

A. basilaris

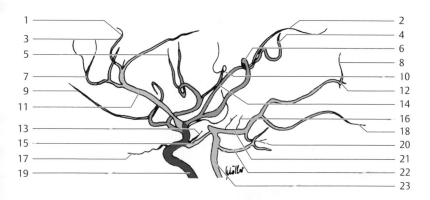

Lateral view

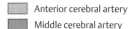 Anterior cerebral artery

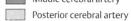 Middle cerebral artery

Posterior cerebral artery

1 Callosomarginal artery
2 Parietal artery
3 Pericallosal artery
4 Artery of angular gyrus
5 Artery of precentral sulcus
6 Middle cerebral artery (opercular part)
7 Polar frontal artery
8 Parieto-occipital artery
9 Medial frontobasal artery
10 Artery of central sulcus
11 Anterior cerebral artery (postcommunicating segment, A2 segment)
12 Medial occipital artery
13 Anterior choroidal artery
14 Middle cerebral artery (M2 segment)
15 Posterior communicating artery
16 Posteromedial central arteries
17 Ophthalmic artery
18 Occipitotemporal branch
19 Internal carotid artery
20 Posterior temporal artery
21 Posterior cerebral artery
22 Superior cerebellar artery
23 Basilar artery

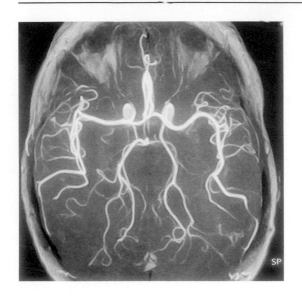

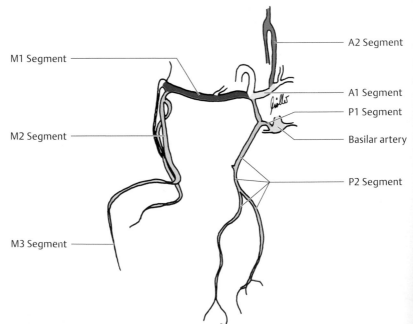

M1 Segment

M2 Segment

M3 Segment

A2 Segment

A1 Segment

P1 Segment

Basilar artery

P2 Segment

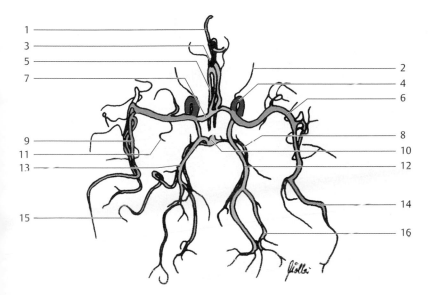

Cranial view

- ▢ Anterior cerebral artery
- ▨ Middle cerebral artery
- ▢ Posterior cerebral artery

1 Anteromedial frontal branch of anterior cerebral artery
2 Ophthalmic artery
3 Anterior cerebral artery (postcommunicating part)
4 Internal carotid artery
5 Anterior communicating artery
6 Middle cerebral artery (sphenoid part)
7 Anterior cerebral artery (precommunicating part)
8 Superior cerebellar artery
9 Middle cerebral artery (insular part)
10 Basilar artery
11 Anterior choroidal artery
12 Left posterior cerebral artery (from internal carotid artery, variant)
13 Right posterior cerebral artery
14 Middle cerebral artery (opercular part)
15 Temporal artery
16 Parieto-occipital artery

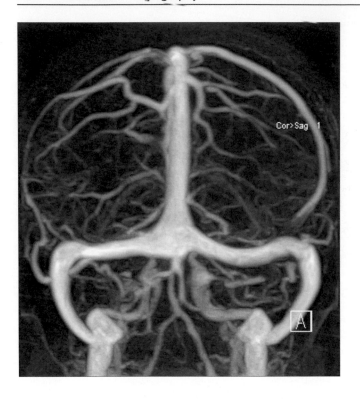

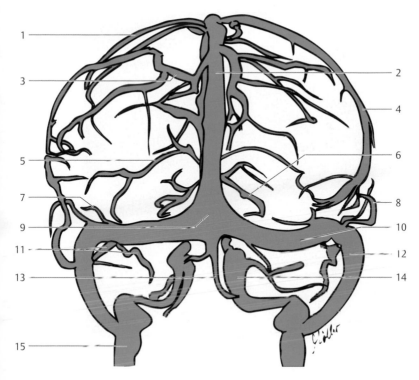

1 Superior cerebral veins
2 Superior sagittal sinus
3 Parietal veins
4 Superior anastomotic vein
   (Trolard)
5 Frontal veins
6 Basal vein
7 Middle cerebral veins (deep
   and superficial)
8 Sphenoparietal sinus

 9 Confluence of sinuses
10 Transverse sinus
11 Superior veins of cerebellar
    hemisphere
12 Sigmoid sinus
13 Inferior veins of cerebellar
    hemisphere
14 Cavernous sinus
15 Internal jugular vein

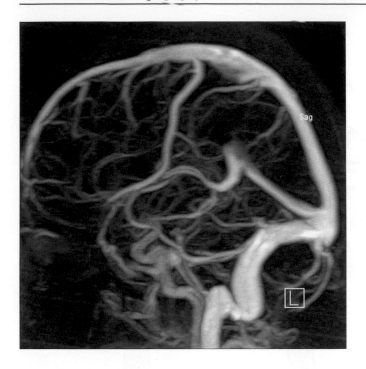

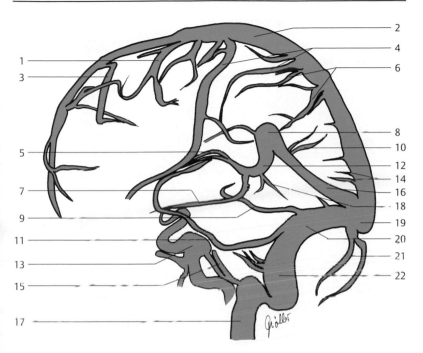

1 Precentral cerebellar veins	12 Great cerebral vein
2 Superior sagittal sinus	13 Cavernous sinus
3 Frontal veins	14 Posterior cerebral veins
4 Superior cerebral veins	15 Inferior petrosal sinus
5 Internal cerebral veins	16 Straight sinus
6 Parietal veins	17 Internal jugular vein
7 Basal vein	18 Superior veins of cerebellar
8 Falcotentorial confluence	hemisphere
of sinuses	19 Confluence of sinuses
9 Inferior anastomotic vein	20 Transverse sinus
(Labbé)	21 Inferior veins of cerebellar
10 Internal occipital vein	hemisphere
11 Superior petrosal sinus	22 Sigmoid sinus

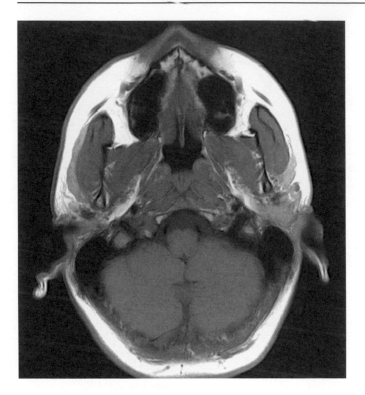

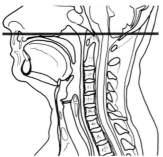

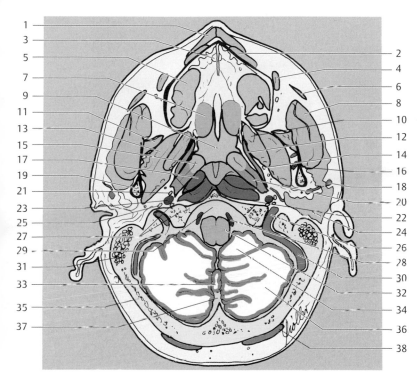

1 Orbicularis oris muscle
2 Levator labii superioris muscle
3 Maxilla (palatine process) and
  incisive canal
4 Levator anguli oris muscle
5 Maxillary sinus
6 Zygomaticus major muscle
7 Soft palate
8 Masseter muscle
9 Nasopharynx
10 Medial pterygoid muscle
11 Temporal muscle
12 Tensor veli palatini muscle
13 Lateral pterygoid muscle
14 Mandibular nerve (V₃)
15 Pharyngotympanic tube (auditory tube) (torus levatorius)
16 Maxillary artery
17 Longus capitis muscle
18 Retromandibular vein
19 Ramus of mandible
20 Levator veli palatini muscle

21 Glossopharyngeal nerve (IX)
22 Occipital bone, basilar part
  (basion)
23 Internal carotid artery
24 Parotid gland
25 Vagus nerve (X)
26 Internal jugular vein
  (superior bulb)
27 Hypoglossal nerve (XII)
28 Vertebral artery
29 Interpeduncular cistern
30 Sigmoid sinus
31 Mastoid cells
32 Medulla oblongata
33 Vermis
34 Tonsil of cerebellum
35 Occipital bone
36 Cerebellar hemisphere
  (posterior lobe)
37 Cisterna magna (posterior
  cerebellomedullary cistern)
38 Semispinalis capitis muscle

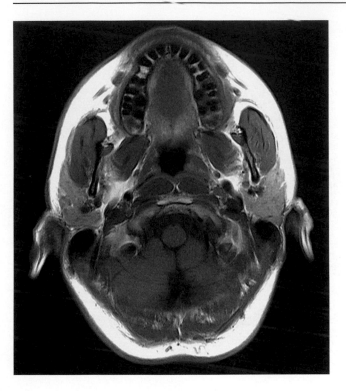

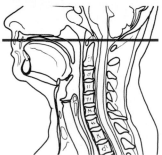

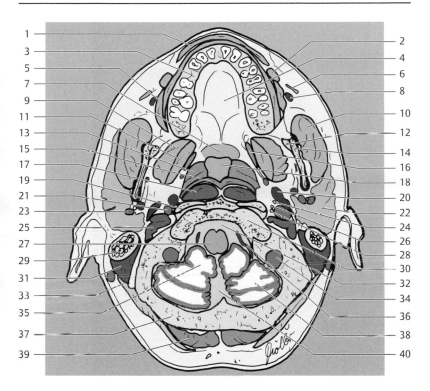

1 Orbicularis oris muscle
2 Levator anguli oris muscle
3 Maxilla (alveolar process)
4 Hard palate
5 Buccinator muscle
6 Zygomaticus muscle
7 Soft palate
8 Facial artery
9 Lateral pterygoid muscle
10 Masseter muscle
11 Medial pterygoid muscle
12 Temporal muscle
13 Levator veli palatini muscle
14 Ramus of mandible
15 Splenius capitis muscle
16 Tensor veli palatini muscle
17 Longus capitis muscle
18 Nasopharynx
19 Anterior arch of atlas
20 Internal carotid artery
21 Internal jugular vein
22 Parotid gland
23 Retromandibular vein
24 Vagus nerve (X)
25 Rectus capitis lateralis muscle
26 Hypoglossal nerve (XII)
27 Medulla oblongata
28 Accessory nerve (XI)
29 Mastoid cells (mastoid process)
30 Occipital bone, basilar part (basion)
31 Digastric muscle (posterior belly)
32 Interpeduncular cistern
33 Splenius capitis muscle
34 Condylar canal with emissary veins
35 Tonsil of cerebellum
36 Vertebral artery
37 Occipital bone
38 Cerebellar hemisphere (posterior lobe)
39 Semispinalis capitis muscle
40 Cisterna magna (posterior cerebellomedullary cistern)

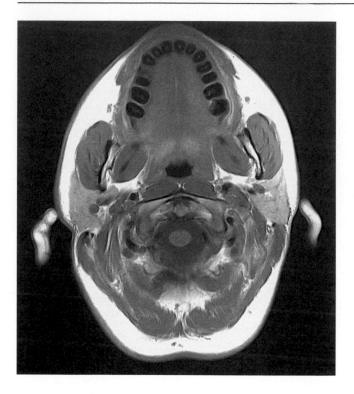

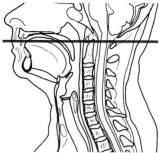

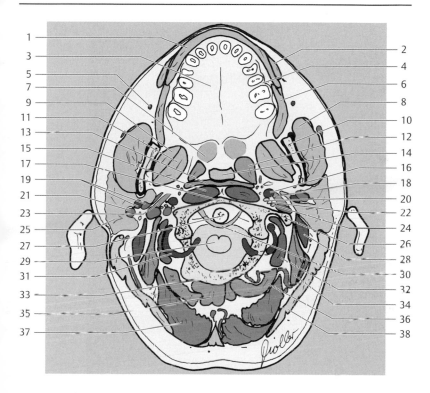

1 Orbicularis oris muscle
2 Levator anguli oris muscle
3 Hard palate
4 Maxilla (alveolar process)
5 Facial artery
6 Buccinator muscle
7 Soft palate
8 Masseter muscle
9 Lateral pterygoid muscle
10 Ramus of mandible
11 Medial pterygoid muscle
12 Tensor veli palatini muscle
13 Superior constrictor muscle of pharynx
14 Pharynx
15 Longus capitis muscle
16 Internal carotid artery
17 Atlas (anterior arch)
18 Glossopharyngeal nerve (IX)
19 Maxillary artery and vein
20 Vagus nerve (X)
21 Retromandibular vein
22 Hypoglossal nerve (XII)
23 Stylopharyngeus muscle
24 Accessory nerve (XI)
25 Parotid gland
26 Atlas, transverse process
27 Dens of axis
28 Digastric muscle (posterior belly)
29 Medulla oblongata
30 Transverse ligament of atlas
31 Vertebral artery
32 Rectus capitis lateralis muscle
33 Atlas, posterior arch
34 Obliquus capitis superior muscle
35 Rectus capitis posterior minor muscle
36 Obliquus capitis inferior muscle
37 Semispinalis capitis muscle
38 Splenius capitis muscle

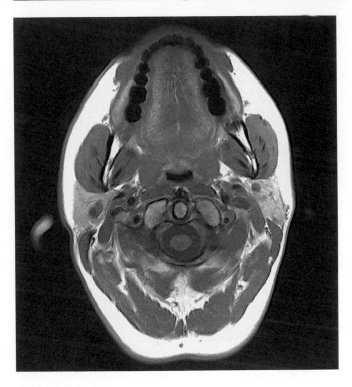

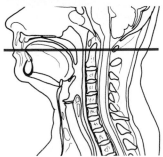

1 Upper lip
2 Incisors (1 and 2 left)
3 Orbicularis oris muscle

4 Canine tooth (3 left)
5 Levator anguli oris muscle
6 Premolar teeth (4 and 5 left)

▶

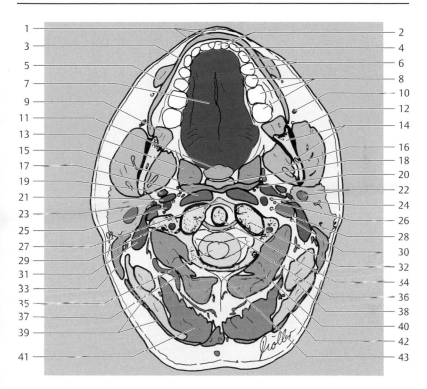

7 Tongue
8 Molar teeth (6, 7 and 8)
9 Buccinator muscle
10 Facial artery
11 Uvula
12 Masseter muscle
13 Tensor veli palatini muscle
14 Ramus of mandible with alveolar canal
15 Superior constrictor muscle of pharynx
16 Medial pterygoid muscle
17 Longus capitis muscle
18 Oropharynx
19 Styloglossus muscle
20 Pharyngeal venous plexus
21 Stylopharyngeus muscle
22 Parotid gland and retromandibular vein
23 Maxillary artery
24 Glossopharyngeal nerve (IX)
25 Internal carotid artery
26 Hypoglossal nerve (XII)
27 Atlas (anterior arch)
28 Vagus nerve (X)
29 Transverse process and foramen transversarium
30 Accessory nerve (XI)
31 Digastric muscle (posterior belly)
32 Atlas, lateral mass
33 Sternocleidomastoid muscle
34 Dens of axis
35 Spinal cord
36 Transverse ligament of atlas
37 Deep cervical veins
38 Longissimus capitis muscle
39 Trapezius muscle
40 Obliquus capitis inferior muscle
41 Semispinalis capitis muscle
42 Splenius capitis muscle
43 Nuchal ligament

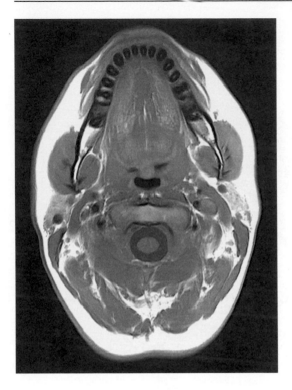

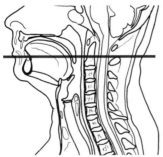

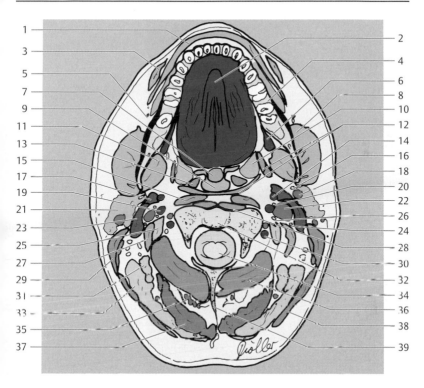

1 Orbicularis oris muscle
2 Tongue (genioglossus muscle)
3 Levator anguli oris muscle
4 Mandible
5 Facial artery
6 Hyoglossus muscle
7 Uvula
8 Masseter muscle
9 Oropharynx
10 Palatine tonsil
11 Medial pterygoid muscle
12 Superior constrictor muscle of pharynx
13 Palatopharyngeus muscle
14 External carotid artery
15 Longus capitis muscle
16 Facial nerve (VII)
17 Stylohyoid muscle, styloglossus muscle
18 Retromandibular vein
19 Internal carotid artery
20 Hypoglossal nerve (XII)
21 Parotid gland
22 Internal jugular vein
23 Digastric muscle (posterior belly)
24 Vagus nerve (X)
25 Longissimus cervicis muscle
26 Accessory nerve (XI)
27 Levator scapulae muscle
28 Longus colli muscle
29 Sternocleidomastoid muscle
30 Vertebral artery
31 Longissimus capitis muscle
32 Axis, body
33 Splenius capitis muscle
34 Spinal cord
35 Deep cervical veins
36 Obliquus capitis inferior muscle
37 Semispinalis capitis muscle
38 Trapezius muscle
39 Nuchal ligament

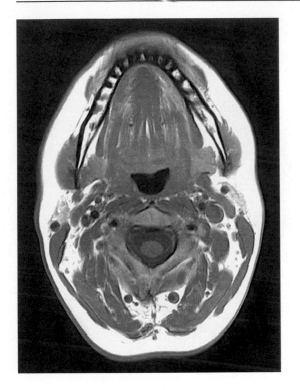

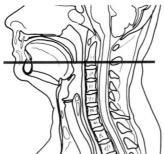

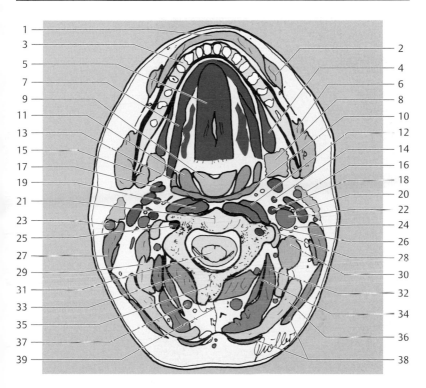

1 Orbicularis oris muscle
2 Depressor anguli oris muscle
3 Mandible
4 Mylohyoid muscle
5 Genioglossus muscle
6 Masseter muscle
7 Hyoglossus muscle
8 Submandibular gland
9 Oropharynx
10 Superior constrictor muscle of pharynx
11 Palatopharyngeus muscle
12 Longus capitis muscle
13 Middle constrictor muscle of pharynx
14 External carotid artery
15 Medial pterygoid muscle
16 Parotid gland
17 Styloglossus muscle and stylohyoid muscle
18 Internal carotid artery
19 Longus colli muscle
20 Hypoglossal nerve (XII)
21 Axis, body
22 Internal jugular vein
23 Retromandibular vein
24 Accessory nerve (XI)
25 Vertebral artery
26 Vagus nerve (X)
27 Sternocleidomastoid muscle
28 Longissimus cervicis muscle
29 Longissimus capitis muscle
30 Levator scapulae muscle
31 Spinal cord
32 Semispinalis capitis muscle
33 Spinalis capitis muscle and multifidus muscle
34 Semispinalis cervicis muscle
35 Spinous process of vertebra
36 Splenius capitis muscle
37 Deep cervical veins
38 Trapezius muscle
39 Nuchal ligament

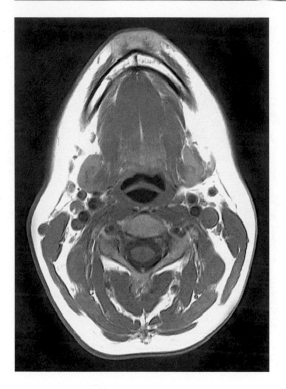

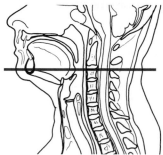

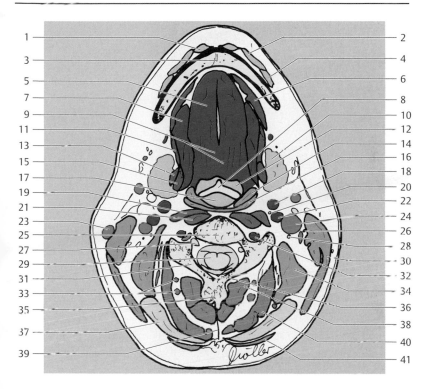

1 Mentalis muscle
2 Depressor anguli oris muscle
3 Mandible
4 Platysma
5 Genioglossus muscle
6 Mylohyoid muscle
7 Hyoglossus muscle
8 Epiglottis
9 Root of tongue
10 Submandibular gland
11 Styloglossus muscle
12 Oropharynx
13 Stylohyoid muscle
14 Palatopharyngeus muscle
15 Digastric muscle (posterior belly)
16 Middle constrictor muscle of pharynx
17 Hypopharynx
18 External carotid artery
19 Longus capitis muscle
20 Superior laryngeal nerve (vagus nerve, X)
21 Longus colli muscle
22 Internal carotid artery
23 External jugular vein
24 Internal jugular vein
25 Cervical vertebra C3 (body)
26 Accessory nerve (XI)
27 Spinal nerve root C4
28 Vagus nerve (X)
29 Spinal cord
30 Sternocleidomastoid muscle
31 Posterior arch of C3
32 Vertebral artery
33 Deep cervical veins
34 Levator scapulae muscle
35 Spinous process
36 Ligamentum flavum
37 Splenius capitis muscle
38 Spinalis cervicis muscle
39 Nuchal ligament
40 Semispinalis capitis muscle
41 Trapezius muscle

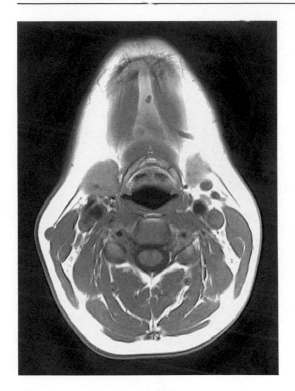

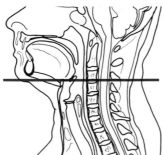

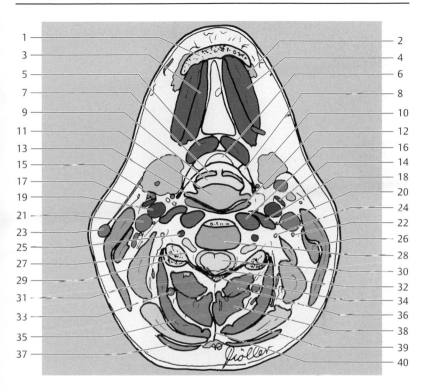

1 Mandible
2 Depressor anguli oris muscle
3 Mylohyoid muscle
4 Digastric muscle (anterior belly)
5 Geniohyoid muscle
6 Hyoid bone (body)
7 Epiglottic vallecula
8 Hyoid bone (greater horn)
9 Epiglottis
10 Submandibular gland
11 Hypopharynx
12 Inferior constrictor muscle of
   pharynx
13 Piriform recess
14 Longus colli muscle
15 Retromandibular vein
16 Superior thyroid artery
17 Platysma
18 Longus capitis muscle
19 Common carotid artery
   (bifurcation)
20 Vagus nerve (X)
21 Internal jugular vein
22 Spinal nerve (C3)
23 External jugular vein
24 Spinal nerve (C2)
25 Vertebral artery
26 Sternocleidomastoid muscle
27 Spinal nerve root (C4)
28 Intervertebral space (C3/C4)
29 Zygapophysial joint
30 Spinal cord
31 Levator scapulae muscle
32 Ligamentum flavum
33 Deep cervical veins
34 Posterior arch of C3 vertebra
35 Semispinalis capitis muscle
36 Spinalis cervicis muscle
37 Trapezius muscle
38 Semispinalis cervicis muscle
39 Splenius capitis muscle
40 Nuchal ligament

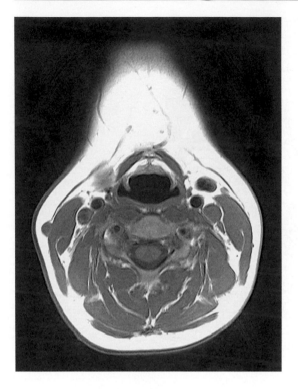

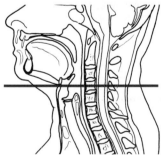

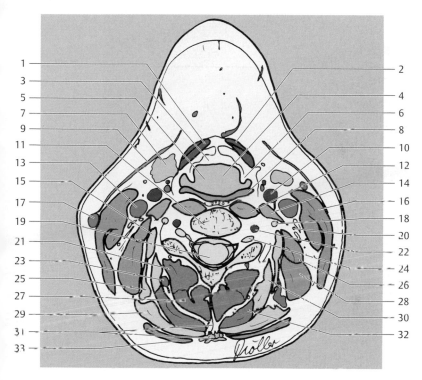

1 Thyrohyoid muscle
2 Sternohyoid muscle
3 Epiglottis (cartilage)
4 Laryngeal vestibule
5 Hypopharynx
6 Ary-epiglottic fold
7 Submandibular gland
8 Inferior constrictor muscle of
   pharynx
9 Platysma
10 Common carotid artery
11 Cervical vertebra C4 (body)
12 Longus colli muscle
13 Internal jugular vein
14 Longus capitis muscle
15 Longissimus capitis muscle
16 Sternocleidomastoid muscle
17 External jugular vein
18 Spinal nerve (C4)
19 Spinal cord
20 Spinal nerve (C3)
21 Spinalis cervicis muscle
22 Vertebral artery
23 Deep cervical veins
24 Spinal nerve root (C5)
25 Longissimus cervicis muscle
26 Middle scalene muscle
27 Semispinalis cervicis muscle
28 Levator scapulae muscle
29 Splenius capitis muscle
30 Splenius cervicis muscle
31 Nuchal ligament
32 Semispinalis capitis muscle
33 Trapezius muscle

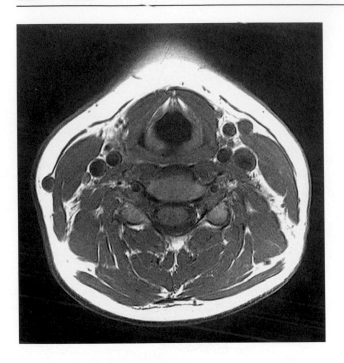

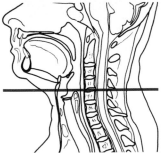

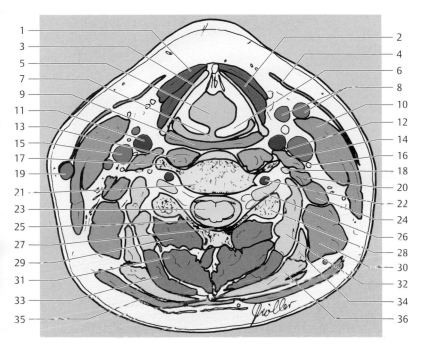

1 Sternohyoid muscle
2 Thyrohyoid muscle
3 Thyroid cartilage (lamina)
4 Platysma
5 Laryngeal vestibule
6 Ary-epiglottic fold
7 Hypopharynx
8 Anterior jugular vein
9 Inferior constrictor muscle of pharynx
10 Sternocleidomastoid muscle
11 Common carotid artery
12 Vagus nerve (X)
13 Longus colli muscle
14 Longus capitis muscle
15 Internal jugular vein
16 Spinal nerve (C4)
17 Transverse process of C5 vertebra
18 Spinal nerve (C5)
19 External jugular vein
20 Middle scalene muscle
21 Cervical vertebra C5 (body)
22 Vertebral artery
23 Spinal cord
24 Posterior scalene muscle
25 Posterior arch of C6 vertebra
26 Spinal nerve root (C6)
27 Ligamentum flavum
28 Inferior articular process of vertebra
29 Spinalis cervicis muscle and multifidus muscle
30 Levator scapulae muscle
31 Semispinalis cervicis muscle
32 Longissimus cervicis muscle
33 Semispinalis capitis muscle
34 Splenius cervicis muscle
35 Trapezius muscle
36 Splenius capitis muscle

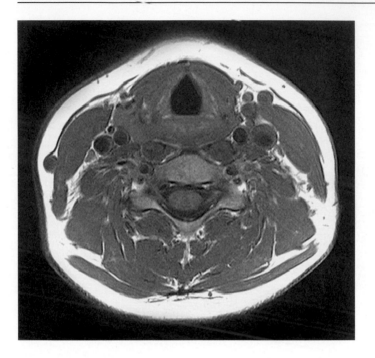

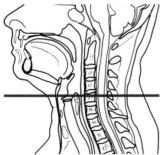

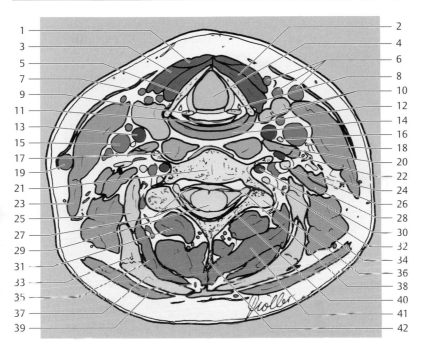

1 Sternohyoid muscle
2 Thyrohyoid muscle
3 Omohyoid muscle
4 Larynx
5 Thyroid cartilage (lamina)
6 Anterior jugular vein
7 Platysma
8 Piriform recess
9 Arytenoid cartilage
10 Thyroid gland
11 Cricoid cartilage
12 Hypopharynx
13 Common carotid artery
14 Inferior constrictor muscle of pharynx
15 Internal jugular vein
16 Vagus nerve (X)
17 Longus colli muscle
18 Phrenic nerve
19 External jugular vein
20 Longus capitis muscle
21 Cervical vertebra C5 (body)

22 Anterior scalene muscle
23 Sternocleidomastoid muscle
24 Posterior scalene muscle
25 Longissimus cervicis muscle
26 Spinal nerve (C4)
27 Anterior and posterior nerve roots
28 Middle scalene muscle
29 Spinal cord
30 Vertebral artery
31 Spinalis cervicis muscle and multifidus muscle
32 Spinal nerve (C5)
33 Splenius cervicis muscle
34 Levator scapulae muscle
35 Semispinalis capitis muscle
36 Inferior articular process of vertebra
37 Splenius capitis muscle
38 Spinal nerve root (C6)
39 Trapezius muscle
40 Posterior arch of C6 vertebra
41 Semispinalis cervicis muscle
42 Spinous process of C6 vertebra

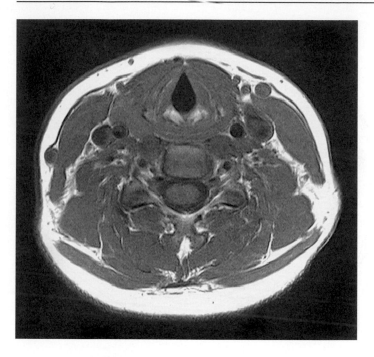

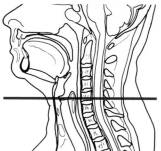

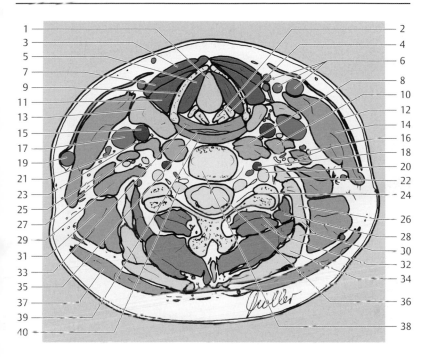

1 Glottis
2 Cricoid cartilage
3 Sternohyoid muscle
4 Arytenoid cartilage
5 Vocalis muscle
6 Anterior jugular vein
7 Omohyoid muscle
8 Longus colli muscle
9 Thyroid cartilage (lamina)
10 Longus capitis muscle
11 Thyrohyoid muscle
12 Platysma
13 Thyroid gland
14 Sternocleidomastoid muscle
15 Common carotid artery
16 Spinal nerves (C4 and C5)
17 Internal jugular vein
18 Vertebral artery
19 External jugular vein
20 Spinal nerve (C6)
21 Phrenic nerve
22 Longissimus capitis muscle
23 Vagus nerve (X)
24 Zygapophysial joint
25 Middle scalene muscle
26 Longissimus cervicis muscle
27 Anterior scalene muscle
28 Semispinalis capitis muscle
29 Posterior scalene muscle
30 Splenius cervicis muscle and splenius capitis muscle
31 Levator scapulae muscle
32 Spinalis cervicis muscle and multifidus muscle
33 Posterior crico-arytenoid muscle
34 Semispinalis cervicis muscle
35 Hypopharynx/esophagus
36 Spinal cord
37 Trapezius muscle
38 Cervical vertebra C5
39 Inferior constrictor muscle of pharynx
40 Nerve root (C7)

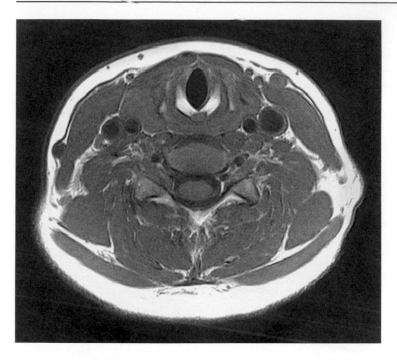

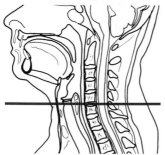

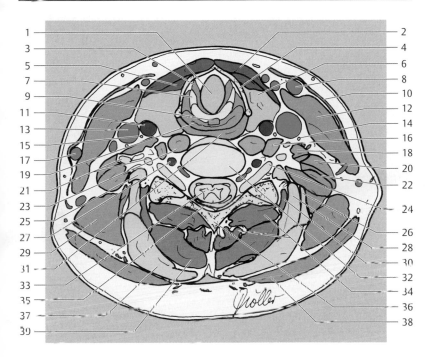

1 Larynx	21 Spinal nerves (C4 and C5)
2 Sternohyoid muscle	22 Posterior scalene muscle
3 Vocalis muscle (vocal cord)	23 Longus colli muscle
4 Thyroid cartilage (lamina)	24 Spinal nerve root (C6)
5 Thyrohyoid muscle	25 Longissimus capitis muscle
6 Thyroid gland	26 Longissimus cervicis muscle
7 Arytenoid cartilage	27 Vertebral artery
8 Anterior jugular vein	28 Splenius cervicis muscle
9 Transverse arytenoid muscle	29 Levator scapulae muscle
10 Platysma	30 Semispinalis capitis muscle
11 Common carotid artery	31 Inferior constrictor muscle of pharynx
12 Sternocleidomastoid muscle	32 Intervertebral space (C5/C6)
13 Internal jugular vein	33 Spinal cord
14 Phrenic muscle	34 Spinalis cervicis muscle and
15 Vagus nerve (X)	multifidus muscle
16 Longus capitis muscle	35 Ligamentum flavum
17 External jugular vein	36 Posterior vertebral arch
18 Anterior scalene muscle	37 Splenius capitis muscle
19 Hypopharynx/esophagus	38 Trapezius muscle
20 Middle scalene muscle	39 Semispinalis cervicis muscle

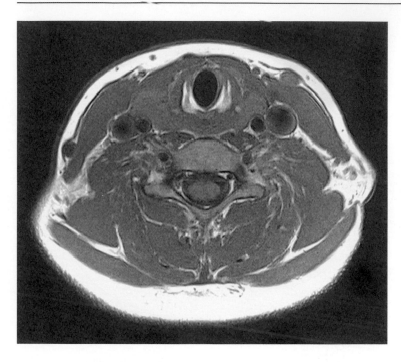

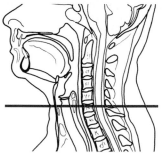

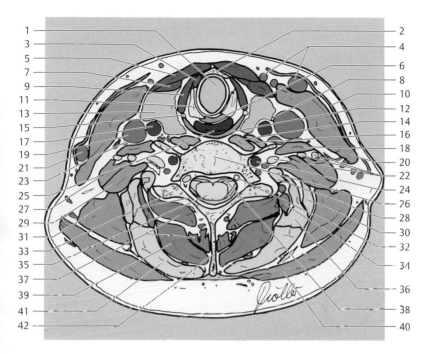

1 Larynx
2 Thyroid cartilage
3 Thyro-arytenoid muscle
4 Anterior jugular vein
5 Sternohyoid muscle
6 Transverse arytenoid muscle
7 Thyrohyoid muscle
8 Vagus nerve (X)
9 Sternothyroid muscle
10 Platysma
11 Cricoid cartilage (lamina)
12 Inferior constrictor muscle of pharynx
13 Thyroid gland
14 Longus colli muscle
15 Thyroid cartilage (inferior horn)
16 Longus capitis muscle
17 Common carotid artery
18 Anterior scalene muscle
19 Internal jugular vein
20 Sternocleidomastoid muscle
21 External jugular vein
22 Spinal nerves (C4, C5, C6)
23 Phrenic nerve
24 Vertebral artery
25 Esophagus
26 Cervical vertebra (C6)
27 Middle scalene muscle
28 Longissimus capitis muscle
29 Posterior scalene muscle
30 Longissimus cervicis muscle
31 Levator scapulae muscle
32 Spinal nerve root (C7)
33 Articular process and posterior arch of C7 vertebra
34 Semispinalis capitis muscle
35 Spinal cord
36 Splenius cervicis muscle
37 Spinalis cervicis muscle and multifidus muscle
38 Anterior and posterior spinal nerve roots (C8)
39 Semispinalis cervicis muscle
40 Trapezius muscle
41 Splenius capitis muscle
42 Spinous process of vertebra

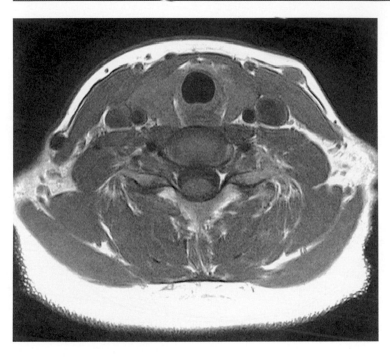

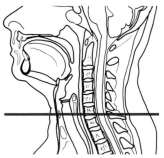

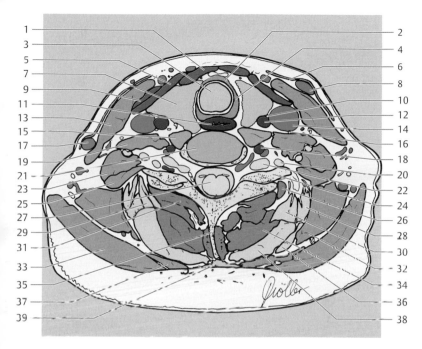

1 Sternohyoid muscle	21 Intervertebral space (C6/C7)
2 Cricoid cartilage (arch)	22 Spinal nerve root (C7)
3 Trachea	23 Middle scalene muscle
4 Cricothyroid muscle	24 Zygapophysial joint (C6/C7)
5 Sternothyroid muscle	25 Posterior scalene muscle
6 Platysma	26 Longissimus capitis muscle
7 Thyroid gland	27 Spinal cord
8 Anterior jugular vein	28 Longissimus cervicis muscle
9 Omohyoid muscle	29 Semispinalis capitis muscle
10 Vagus nerve (X)	30 Splenius cervicis muscle
11 Esophagus	31 Spinalis cervicis muscle and multifidus muscle
12 Common carotid artery	32 Levator scapulae muscle
13 Sternocleidomastoid muscle	33 Trapezius muscle
14 Internal jugular vein	34 Semispinalis cervicis muscle
15 Longus colli muscle	35 Spinous process of vertebra
16 Phrenic muscle	36 Serratus posterior superior muscle
17 External jugular vein	37 Rhomboid minor muscle
18 Vertebral artery	38 Splenius capitis muscle
19 Anterior scalene muscle	39 Nuchal ligament
20 Spinal nerves (C4, C5, and C6)	

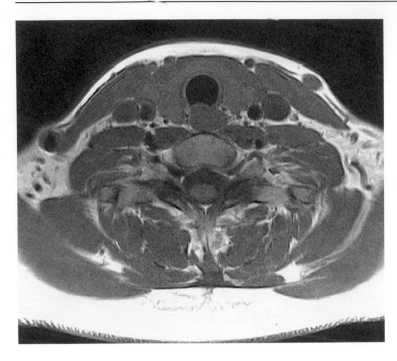

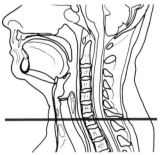

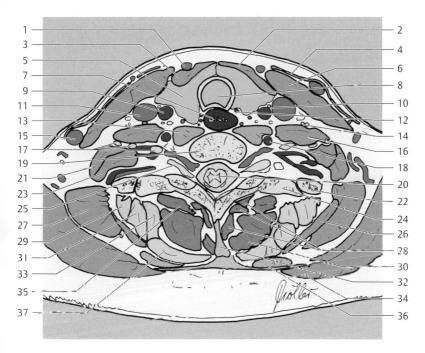

1 Anterior jugular vein
2 Sternohyoid muscle
3 Sternothyroid muscle
4 Platysma
5 Thyroid gland
6 Sternocleidomastoid muscle
7 Esophagus
8 Trachea
9 Common carotid artery
10 Vagus nerve (X)
11 Internal jugular vein
12 Inferior thyroid artery
13 Longus colli muscle
14 Phrenic nerve
15 External jugular vein
16 Anterior scalene muscle
17 Spinal nerves (C5, C6, and C7)
18 Vertebral artery
19 Cervical vertebra (C7)

20 Spinal cord
21 Middle scalene muscle
22 First rib
23 Posterior scalene muscle
24 Transverse process of vertebra
25 Spinal nerve root (C8)
26 Serratus posterior superior muscle
27 Levator scapulae muscle
28 Spinalis cervicis muscle and
   multifidus muscle
29 Iliocostalis cervicis muscle
30 Semispinalis cervicis muscle
31 Longissimus cervicis muscle
32 Interspinous ligament
33 Splenius cervicis muscle
34 Trapezius muscle
35 Semispinalis capitis muscle
36 Rhomboid minor muscle
37 Splenius capitis muscle

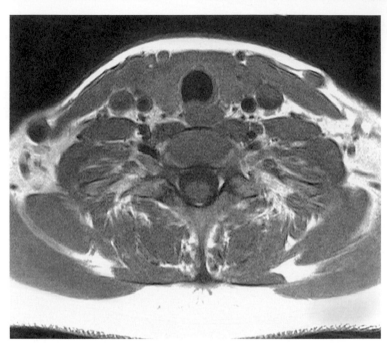

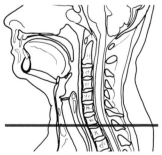

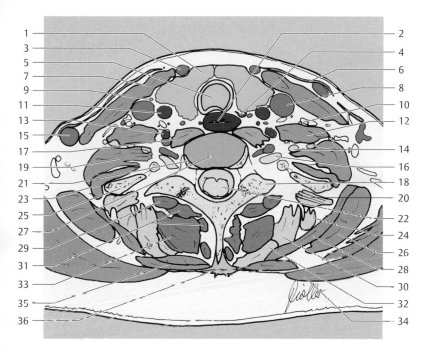

1 Sternohyoid muscle
2 Esophagus
3 Anterior jugular vein and thyroid gland
4 Inferior thyroid artery
5 Trachea
6 Platysma
7 Sternocleidomastoid muscle
8 Internal jugular vein
9 Vagus nerve (X)
10 Phrenic nerve
11 Common carotid artery
12 Anterior scalene muscle
13 Vertebral artery
14 Spinal nerves (C5, C6, and C7)
15 External jugular vein
16 Spinal nerve root (C8)
17 Longus colli muscle
18 Transverse process of T1 vertebra
19 Middle scalene muscle

20 Intercostal muscles
21 Superior posterior margin of T1 vertebra
22 Spinal cord
23 Posterior scalene muscle
24 Iliocostalis cervicis muscle
25 First rib
26 Levator scapulae muscle
27 Intervertebral space (C7/T1)
28 Serratus posterior superior muscle
29 Semispinalis capitis muscle
30 Splenius cervicis muscle
31 Spinalis cervicis muscle and multifidus muscle
32 Splenius capitis muscle
33 Semispinalis cervicis muscle
34 Trapezius muscle
35 Rhomboid minor muscle
36 Interspinous ligament

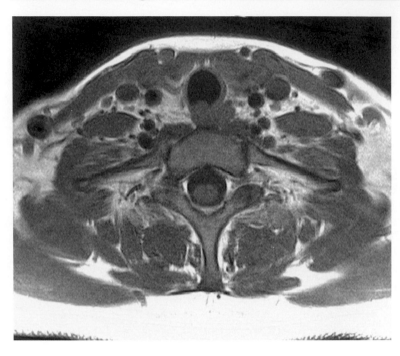

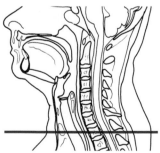

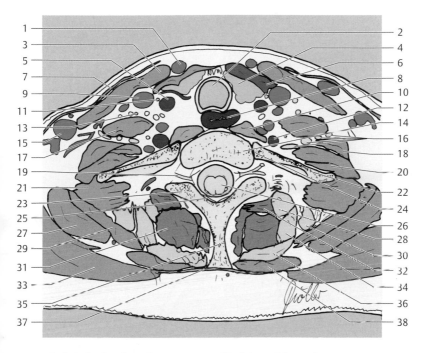

1 Anterior jugular vein
2 Trachea
3 Sternocleidomastoid muscle
4 Thyroid gland
5 Common carotid artery
6 Sternohyoid muscle
7 Platysma
8 Esophagus
9 Internal jugular vein
10 Longus colli muscle
11 Vagus nerve (X)
12 Vertebral artery
13 Phrenic nerve
14 Vertebra (T1)
15 External jugular vein
16 Cervical plexus (C5 to C8)
17 Anterior scalene muscle
18 Middle scalene muscle
19 Spinal nerve root (T1)
20 Posterior scalene muscle

21 Intercostal muscles
22 First rib
23 Transverse process of T1 vertebra
24 Costovertebral joint
25 Ligamentum flavum
26 Spinal cord
27 Levator scapulae muscle
28 Semispinalis capitis muscle
29 Serratus posterior superior muscle
30 Iliocostalis cervicis muscle
31 Semispinalis cervicis muscle
32 Spinalis cervicis muscle and
   multifidus muscle
33 Trapezius muscle
34 Splenius cervicis muscle
35 Spinous process of vertebra
36 Splenius capitis muscle
37 Interspinous ligament
38 Rhomboid minor muscle

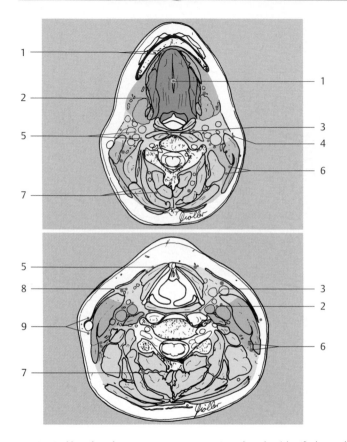

Cervical lymph nodes

1 Submental lymph nodes
2 Submandibular lymph nodes
3 Retropharyngeal lymph nodes
4 Pre-auricular lymph nodes
5 Superior jugular group of lymph nodes
6 Deep cervical lymph nodes
7 Nuchal lymph nodes
8 Anterior jugular lymph nodes
9 Superficial cervical lymph nodes

Lymph nodes (classified according to levels)

Level 1a (submental lymph nodes between digastric muscles)

Level 1b (submandibular lymph nodes)

Level 2a (lymph nodes anterior, medial or lateral to the internal jugular vein)

Level 2b (lymph nodes dorsal to the internal jugular vein and separated from the vein by a lamella of fat)

Level 3 (lymph nodes along the jugular vein)

Level 5a (lymph nodes in the posterior triangle, upper level = above arch of cricoid cartilage)

Level 6 (upper visceral lymph nodes: ventral between the carotid arteries)

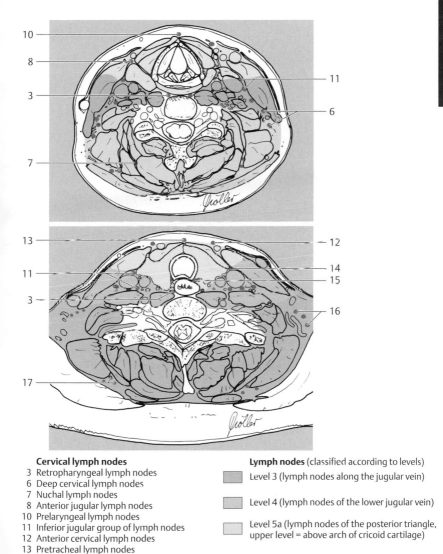

Cervical lymph nodes
3 Retropharyngeal lymph nodes
6 Deep cervical lymph nodes
7 Nuchal lymph nodes
8 Anterior jugular lymph nodes
10 Prelaryngeal lymph nodes
11 Inferior jugular group of lymph nodes
12 Anterior cervical lymph nodes
13 Pretracheal lymph nodes
14 Thyroid lymph nodes
15 Paratracheal lymph nodes
16 Supraclavicular lymph nodes
17 Superficial cervical lymph nodes

Lymph nodes (classified according to levels)

Level 3 (lymph nodes along the jugular vein)

Level 4 (lymph nodes of the lower jugular vein)

Level 5a (lymph nodes of the posterior triangle, upper level = above arch of cricoid cartilage)

Level 5b (lymph nodes of the posterior triangle, lower level = below arch of cricoid cartilage)

Level 6 (upper visceral lymph nodes: ventral between the carotid arteries)

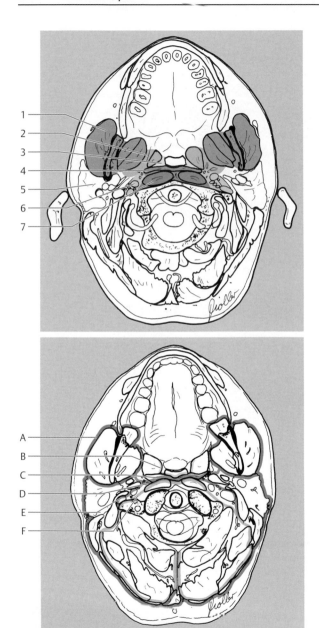

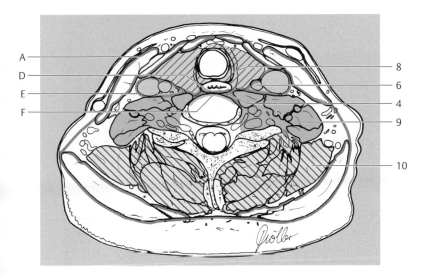

Cervical spaces

1 Masticatory space (chewing muscles, ramus and body of mandible, inferior alveolar nerve, maxillary artery, pterygoid plexus, lingual nerve)

2 Parapharyngeal space (trigeminal nerve, pharyngeal artery)

3 Superficial mucosal space (submucosal salivary glands, lymphatic tissue)

4 Retropharyngeal space

5 Parotid space (parotid gland, facial nerve, external carotid artery, retromandibular vein)

6 Carotid space (carotid artery, jugular vein, cranial nerves IX–XII, sympathetic trunk)

7 Prevertebral space (prevertebral and paraspinal muscles, phrenic nerve)

8 Visceral space (thyroid gland, paratracheal space)

9 Perivertebral space (prevertebral part)

10 Perivertebral space (paraspinal part)

Cervical fasciae

A Superficial cervical fascia (fascia colli superficialis)

B Pharyngobasilar fascia

C Middle layer of deep cervical fascia (pretracheal layer)

D Intercarotid fascia

E Carotid sheath

F Deep layer of deep cervical fascia (prevertebral layer)

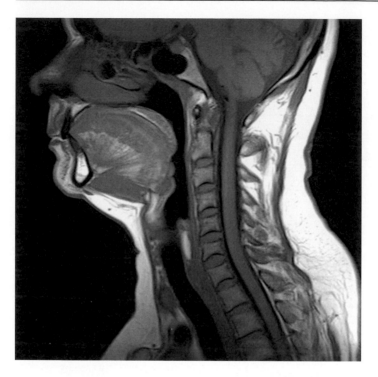

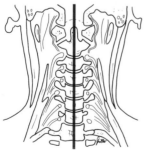

1 Palatine tonsil
2 Foramen magnum
3 Vomer
4 Anterior longitudinal ligament
5 Nasopharynx and longus colli
  muscle

6 Apical ligament of dens
7 Hard palate
8 Tectorial membrane
9 Incisive canal
10 Posterior atlanto-occipital membrane
11 Orbicularis oris muscle   ▶

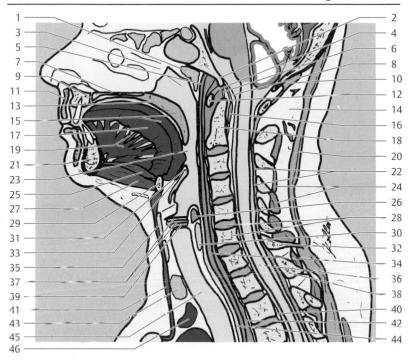

12 Anterior arch of atlas
13 Soft palate
14 Suboccipital fatty tissue
15 Superior longitudinal muscle
   of tongue and oral cavity
16 Transverse ligament of atlas
   (of cruciform ligament of atlas)
17 Transverse muscle of tongue
18 Dens of axis (C2)
19 Genioglossus muscle and
   lingual septum
20 Nuchal ligament
21 Mandible
22 Ligamentum flavum
23 Oropharynx
24 Interspinales muscles
25 Geniohyoid muscle
26 Transverse and oblique
   arytenoid muscles
27 Mylohyoid muscle
28 Vertebra C6 and intervertebral
   disc

29 Hyoid bone
30 Larynx (lamina)
31 Epiglottis
32 Spinous process of C7
33 Epiglottic vallecula
34 Inferior constrictor muscle of
   pharynx
35 Thyroid cartilage
36 Spinal cord
37 Vestibular ligament (false vocal cord)
   and laryngeal ventricle (ventricle of
   Morgagni)
38 Spinous process
39 Vocal ligament (true vocal cord)
40 Posterior longitudinal ligament
41 Sternothyroid muscle
42 Anterior longitudinal ligament
43 Thyroid gland
44 Esophagus
45 Trachea
46 Brachiocephalic artery

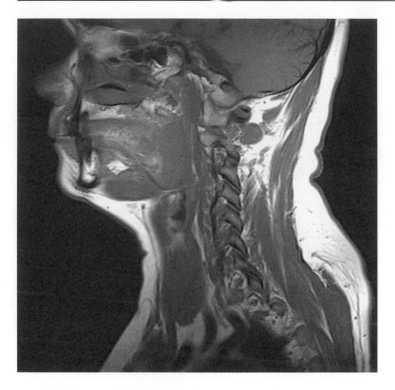

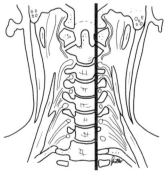

1 Levator veli palatini muscle
2 Semispinalis capitis muscle
3 Medial pterygoid muscle
4 Atlas (lateral mass)
5 Longus capitis muscle

6 Rectus capitis posterior minor muscle
7 Maxilla
8 Rectus capitis posterior major muscle
9 Orbicularis oris muscle
10 Inferior oblique muscle

►

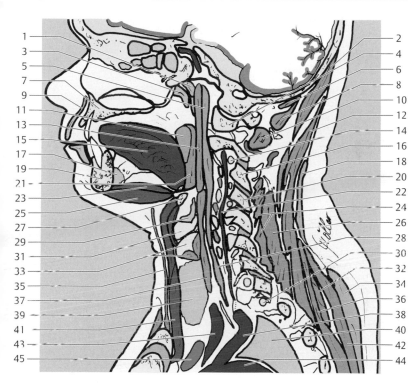

11 Palatine tonsil
12 Splenius capitis muscle
13 Superior constrictor muscle of pharynx
14 Spinal nerve root (C3)
15 Tongue
16 Inferior articular process
17 Sublingual gland
18 Trapezius muscle (descending part)
19 Mandible
20 Superior articular process
21 Palatopharyngeus muscle
22 Vertebral artery
23 Mylohyoid muscle
24 Multifidus muscle
25 Digastric muscle (anterior belly)
26 Semispinalis cervicis muscle
27 Hyoid bone
28 Longus colli muscle
29 Pharynx and epiglottic vallecula
30 Spinal nerve root (T1)
31 Thyroid cartilage
32 Serratus posterior superior muscle
33 Cricoid cartilage and crico-arytaenoid muscle
34 Trapezius muscle
35 Platysma
36 Splenius cervicis muscle
37 Inferior constrictor muscle of pharynx
38 Left subclavian artery
39 Thyroid gland
40 Left lung
41 Sternohyoid muscle
42 Rhomboid (major and minor) muscles
43 Common carotid artery
44 Aortic arch
45 Left brachiocephalic vein

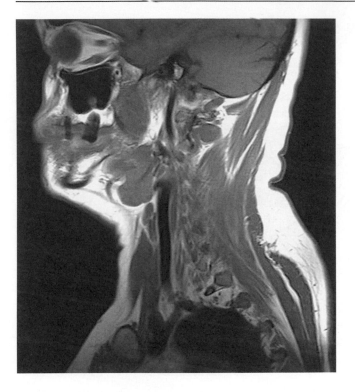

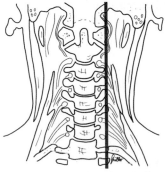

1 Maxillary sinus
2 Internal carotid artery (carotid siphon)
3 Medial pterygoid muscle

4 Mandibular nerve
5 Levator labii superioris muscle
6 Pharyngotympanic tube (auditory tube)
7 Digastric muscle ▶

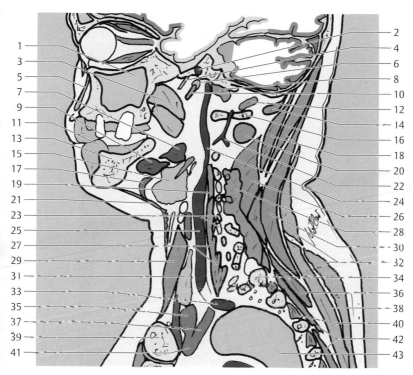

8 Rectus capitis lateralis muscle
9 Mylohyoid muscle
10 Tensor veli palatini muscle
11 Orbicularis oris muscle
12 Obliquus capitis superior muscle
13 Mandible
14 Rectus capitis posterior major muscle
15 Submandibular gland
16 Atlas (transverse process)
17 Facial vein
18 Semispinalis capitis muscle
19 Longus colli muscle
20 Obliquus capitis inferior muscle
21 Platysma
22 Vertebral artery
23 Transverse processes and spinal nerve roots
24 Internal carotid artery

25 Common carotid artery
26 Semispinalis cervicis muscle
27 Scalenus anterior muscle
28 Scalenus posterior muscle
29 Sternocleidomastoid muscle
30 Splenius capitis muscle
31 Thyroid gland
32 Trapezius muscle
33 Subclavian artery
34 First rib
35 Internal jugular vein
36 Semispinalis cervicis muscle
37 Subclavian vein (left)
38 Rhomboid (major and minor) muscle
39 Clavicle
40 Interspinales muscles
41 Brachiocephalic vein (left)
42 Serratus anterior muscle
43 Lung (left)

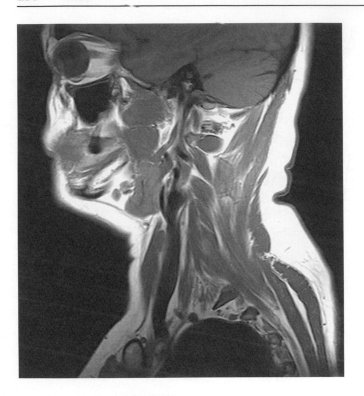

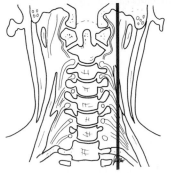

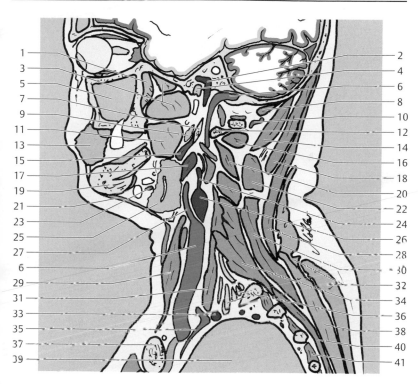

1 Temporal muscle
2 Internal carotid artery (siphon)
3 Lateral pterygoid muscle
4 Pharyngotympanic tube (auditory tube)
5 Maxillary sinus
6 Internal jugular vein
7 Styloid process
8 Rectus capitis posterior minor muscle
9 Parotid gland
10 Deep cervical veins
11 Medial pterygoid muscle
12 Atlas (transverse process)
13 Buccinator muscle
14 Rectus capitis posterior major muscle
15 Stylohyoid muscle
16 Obliquus capitis muscle
17 Digastric muscle
18 Semispinalis capitis muscle
19 Mandible

20 Levator scapulae muscle
21 Platysma
22 Semispinalis cervicis muscle
23 Facial vein
24 External carotid artery
25 Submandibular gland
26 Common carotid artery
27 External jugular vein
28 Splenius capitis muscle
29 Sternocleidomastoid muscle
30 Semispinalis cervicis muscle
31 Scalenus medius muscle
32 Trapezius muscle
33 Subclavian artery (left)
34 Scalenus posterior muscle
35 Subclavian vein (left)
36 Brachial plexus
37 Clavicle
38 Rhomboid (major and minor) muscles
39 Lung (left)
40 Multifidus muscle
41 Interspinales muscles

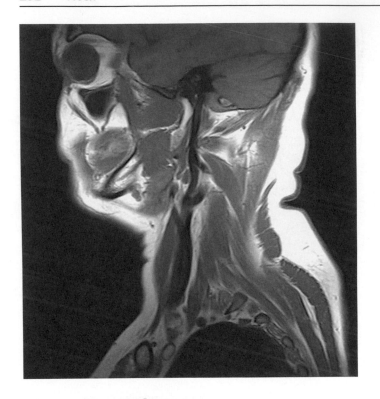

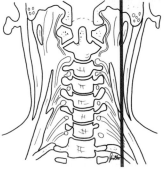

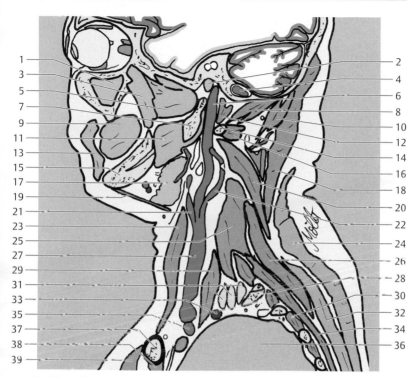

1 Maxillary sinus
2 External acoustic meatus
3 Temporal muscle
4 Sigmoid sinus
5 Lateral pterygoid muscle
6 Internal jugular vein
7 Ramus of the mandible
8 Obliquus capitis posterior major and minor muscles
9 Buccinator muscle
10 Semispinalis capitis muscle
11 Medial pterygoid muscle
12 Rectus capitis lateralis muscle
13 Orbicularis oris muscle
14 Transverse process of cervical vertebra C1
15 Mandible
16 Obliquus capitis superior muscle
17 Submandibular gland
18 Splenius capitis muscle
19 Platysma
20 Levator scapulae muscle
21 Common facial vein
22 Cervical veins
23 Sternocleidomastoid muscle
24 Trapezius muscle
25 Scalenus medius muscle
26 Semispinalis cervicis muscle
27 Internal jugular vein
28 First rib
29 Scalenus anterior muscle
30 Interspinales muscles
31 Brachial plexus
32 Rhomboid (major and minor) muscle
33 Subclavian artery (left)
34 Serratus anterior muscle
35 Subclavian vein (left)
36 Left Lung
37 Clavicle
38 Subclavian muscle
39 Pectoralis major muscle

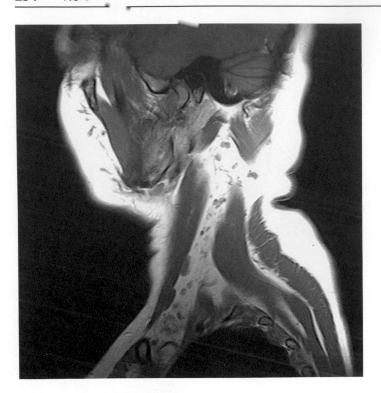

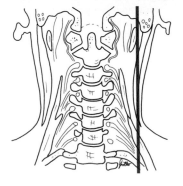

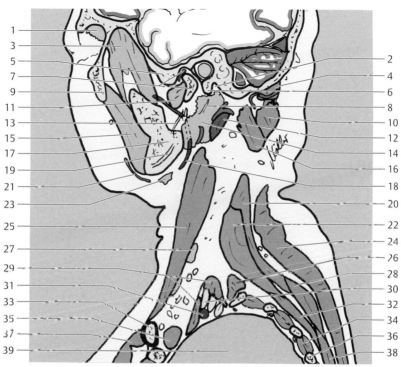

1 Lacrimal gland
2 Stylomastoid foramen
3 Temporal muscle
4 Obliquus capitis superior muscle
5 Articular tubercle
6 Styloid process
7 Head of mandible and articular disc
8 Facial nerve (VII)
9 Zygomatic bone
10 Splenius capitis muscle
11 Lateral pterygoid muscle
12 Digastric muscle (posterior belly)
13 Inferior alveolar nerve
14 Parotid gland
15 Masseter muscle
16 Semispinalis capitis muscle
17 Mandible
18 External carotid artery
19 Mandibular canal
20 Levator scapulae muscle
21 Platysma
22 Scalenus posterior muscle
23 Submandibular gland
24 Trapezius muscle
25 Sternocleidomastoid muscle
26 Scalenus medius muscle
27 Lymph nodes
28 Rhomboid minor muscle
29 Scalenus anterior muscle
30 Brachial plexus
31 Subclavian artery (left)
32 Serratus anterior muscle
33 Clavicle
34 Interspinales muscles
35 Subclavian muscle
36 Fourth rib
37 Pectoralis major muscle
38 Rhomboid major muscle
39 Lung (left)

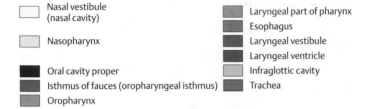

Nasal vestibule (nasal cavity)

Nasopharynx

Oral cavity proper

Isthmus of fauces (oropharyngeal isthmus)

Oropharynx

Laryngeal part of pharynx

Esophagus

Laryngeal vestibule

Laryngeal ventricle

Infraglottic cavity

Trachea

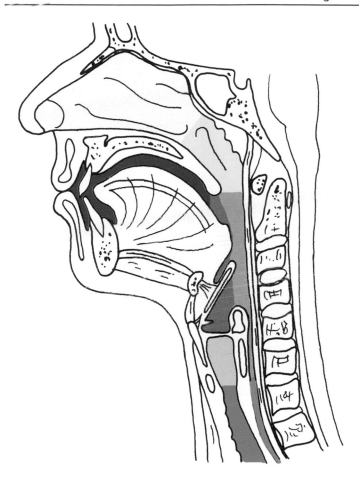

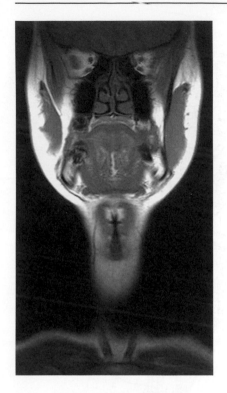

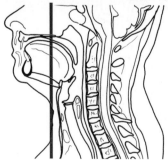

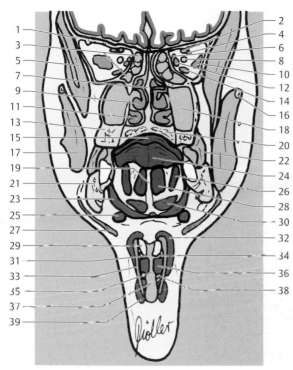

1   Sphenoidal bone (lesser wing)
2   Levator palpebrae superioris
    muscle
3   Ethmoidal cells (anterior)
4   Superior rectus muscle
5   Temporal muscle
6   Superior oblique muscle
7   Nasal septum
8   Optic nerve (II)
9   Middle nasal concha
10 Lateral rectus muscle
11 Inferior nasal concha
12 Medial rectus muscle
13 Mandible
14 Inferior rectus muscle
15 Longitudinal muscle of tongue
16 Zygomatic bone (temporal process)
17 Masseter muscle
18 Maxillary sinus
19 Lingual septum
20 Hard palate
21 Mandible
22 Buccinator muscle
23 Mylohyoid muscle
24 Transverse muscle of tongue
25 Digastric muscle (anterior belly)
26 Hyoglossus muscle
27 Platysma
28 Genioglossus muscle
29 Vestibular fold
30 Geniohyoid muscle
31 Glottis
32 Thyrohyoid muscle
33 Thyroid cartilage
34 Laryngeal ventricle
35 Infraglottic cavity
36 Vocalis muscle
37 Trachea
38 Cricoid cartilage
39 Sternohyoid muscle

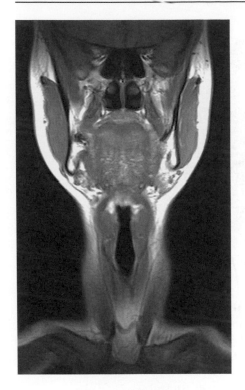

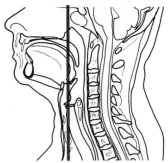

1 Superior orbital fissure
2 Optic nerve (II)
3 Sphenoidal bone (lesser wing)
4 Trochlear nerve (IV)

5 Temporal bone
6 Frontal nerve
7 Foramen rotundum with maxillary nerve
   (V_2)   ▶

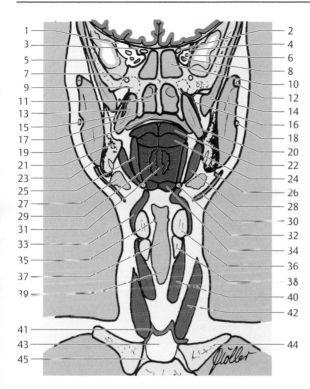

8 Superior ophthalmic vein
9 Pterygopalatine fossa
10 Sphenoidal sinus
11 Dorsal nasal cavity and nasal septum
12 Zygomatic bone (temporal process)
13 Pterygoid fossa
14 Temporal muscle
15 Lateral pterygoid process
16 Maxillary artery
17 Medial pterygoid process
18 Facial nerve (VII)
19 Soft palate
20 Medial pterygoid muscle
21 Mandible (ramus)
22 Longitudinal muscle of tongue
23 Masseter muscle
24 Transverse muscle of tongue
25 Hyoglossus muscle

26 Facial artery
27 Submandibular gland
28 Mylohyoid muscle
29 Vertical muscle of tongue
30 Platysma
31 Lingual septum
32 Hyoid bone
33 Thyrohyoid muscle
34 Geniohyoid muscle
35 Laryngeal ventricle
36 Thyroid cartilage
37 Infraglottic cavity
38 Cricoid cartilage
39 Larynx
40 Cricothyroid muscle
41 Anterior jugular vein
42 Sternohyoid muscle
43 Suprasternal space
44 Clavicle
45 Sternoclavicular joint

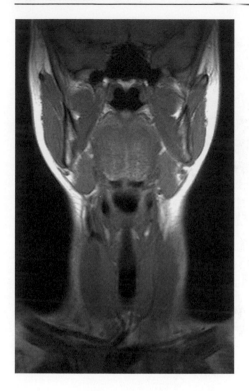

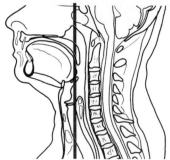

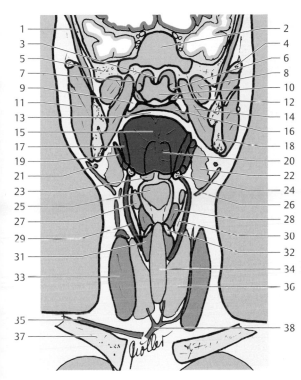

1 Temporal muscle
2 Sphenoidal sinus
3 Vomer
4 Zygomatic bone (temporal process)
5 Sphenoidal bone (greater wing)
6 Pharyngotympanic tube (auditory tube) (cartilage)
7 Lateral and medial plates of pterygoid process
8 Lateral pterygoid muscle
9 Peripharyngeal space
10 Nasopharynx
11 Masseter muscle
12 Levator veli palatini muscle
13 Oropharynx
14 Medial pterygoid muscle
15 Transverse muscle of tongue
16 Soft palate
17 Hyoglossus muscle
18 Mandible
19 Digastric muscle
20 Genioglossus muscle
21 Facial artery
22 Submandibular gland
23 Epiglottic vallecula
24 Hyoid bone (greater horn)
25 Laryngeal vestibule
26 Platysma
27 Piriform recess
28 Ary-epiglottic muscle with ary-epiglottic fold
29 Omohyoid muscle
30 Thyroid cartilage
31 Thyro-arytenoid muscle
32 Arytenoid cartilage
33 Sternocleidomastoid muscle
34 Trachea
35 Anterior jugular vein
36 Thyroid gland
37 Clavicle
38 Inferior thyroid veins

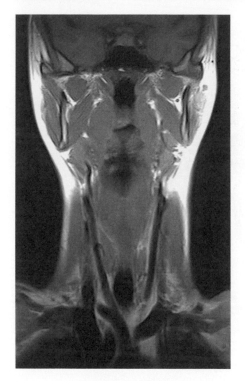

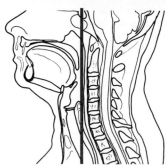

1 Temporal muscle
2 Sphenoidal sinus
3 Sphenoidal bone (greater wing)
4 Oropharynx

5 Zygomatic bone
6 Pharyngotympanic tube (auditory tube)
   (cartilage)
7 Pharyngeal tonsil ▶

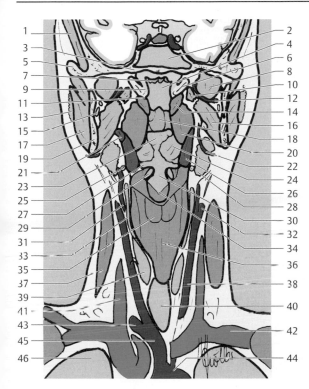

8 Lateral pterygoid muscle
9 Torus tubarius
10 Tensor veli palatini muscle
11 Pharyngeal opening of auditory tube
12 Maxillary artery
13 Parotid gland
14 Levator veli palatini muscle
15 Inferior alveolar nerve
16 Medial pterygoid muscle
17 Masseter muscle
18 Soft palate and uvula
19 Ramus of mandible
20 Palatopharyngeus muscle
21 Styloglossus muscle
22 Facial artery
23 Oropharynx
24 Palatine tonsil
25 Hyoid bone
26 Digastric muscle

27 Epiglottic vallecula
28 Submandibular gland
29 Epiglottis
30 Laryngeal inlet
31 External carotid artery
32 Internal carotid artery
33 Thyroid cartilage
34 Interarytenoid notch
35 Posterior crico-arytenoid muscle
36 Middle constrictor muscle of pharynx
37 Sternocleidomastoid muscle
38 Common carotid artery
39 Thyroid gland
40 Trachea
41 Internal jugular vein
42 Subclavian vein
43 Subclavian artery (right)
44 Aorta
45 Brachiocephalic trunk
46 Lung (right)

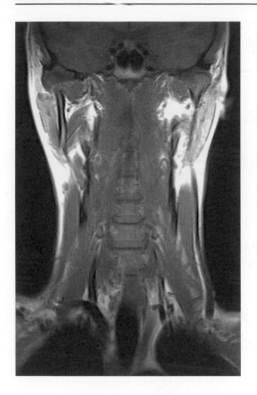

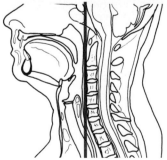

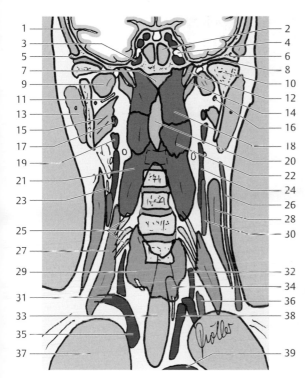

1 Temporal muscle
2 Sphenoidal sinus
3 Internal carotid artery (siphon)
4 Trigeminal cavity
5 Zygomatic process
6 Socket of temporomandibular joint (temporal bone)
7 Nasopharynx
8 Articular disc
9 Lateral pterygoid muscle
10 Head of mandible
11 Lingual nerve
12 Pharyngotympanic tube (auditory tube)
13 Parotid gland
14 Levator veli palatini muscle
15 Medial pterygoid muscle
16 Maxillary artery
17 Stylopharyngeus muscle
18 Longus capitis muscle
19 Digastric muscle
20 Oropharynx
21 Longus colli muscle
22 Longus capitis muscle
23 Vagus nerve (X)
24 Internal carotid artery
25 Spinal nerve roots (cervical plexus)
26 External jugular vein
27 Anterior scalene muscle
28 Sternocleidomastoid muscle
29 Inferior constrictor muscle of pharynx
30 Internal jugular vein
31 Subclavian artery
32 Vertebral artery
33 Trachea
34 Vertebral vein
35 Brachiocephalic trunk
36 Vertebral vein
37 Lung (right)
38 Common carotid artery
39 Aortic arch

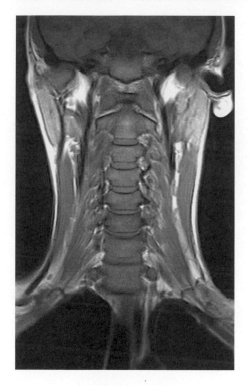

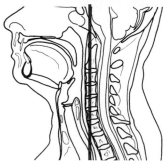

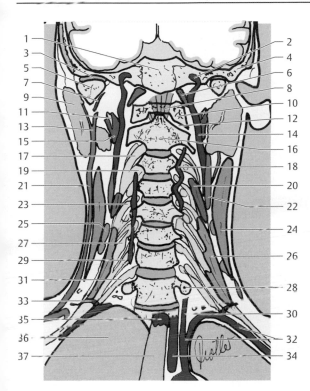

1 Clivus
2 Internal carotid artery (siphon)
3 Articular disc
4 Petrous part of temporal bone
5 Head of mandible
6 Rectus capitis anterior muscle
7 Maxillary artery
8 Anterior atlanto-occipital
   membrane
9 Parotid gland
10 Atlas (lateral mass)
11 Styloid process
12 Atlanto-axial joint
13 Retromandibular vein
14 Internal carotid artery
15 Digastric muscle
16 Axis
17 Spinal nerve root C3
18 Vertebral artery
19 Spinal nerve root C4
20 Longus colli muscle
21 External jugular vein
22 Internal jugular vein
23 Spinal nerve root C5
24 Sternocleidomastoid muscle
25 Lymph nodes
26 Anterior scalene muscle
27 Spinal nerve root C6
28 Costal process
29 Spinal nerve root C7
30 Vertebral artery (left)
31 Spinal nerve root C8
32 Subclavian artery
33 Suprascapular artery
34 Internal carotid artery
35 Esophagus
36 Lung (right)
37 Trachea

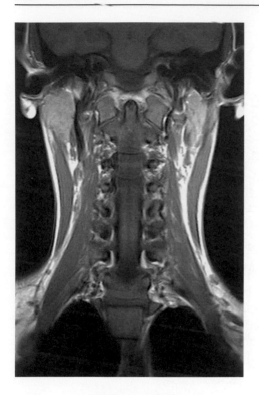

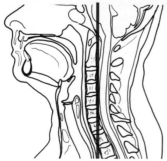

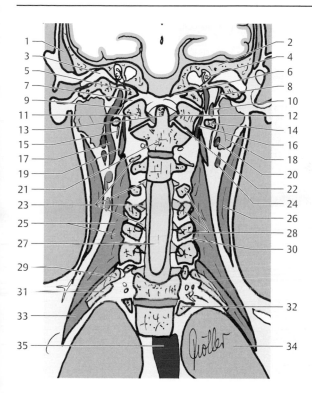

1 Temporal muscle
2 Petrous part of temporal bone
3 External acoustic meatus
4 Tympanic cavity
5 Occipital condyle
6 Clivus
7 Atlanto-occipital joint
8 Styloid process
9 Accessory nerve (XI) and
  hypoglossal nerve (XII)
10 Stylopharyngeus muscle
11 Atlas (lateral mass)
12 Alar ligaments
13 Dens of axis
14 Atlas (transverse process)
15 Vagus nerve (X)
16 Vertebral artery
17 Internal jugular vein
18 Parotid gland
19 Obliquus capitis inferior muscle
20 Stylohyoid muscle
21 Axis (body)
22 Atlanto-axial joint
23 Spinal nerve roots C3–C6
24 Digastric muscle
25 Middle scalene muscle
26 Sternocleidomastoid muscle
27 Spinal cord
28 Articular processes C4–C6
29 Spinal nerve root C8
30 Zygapophysial joint
31 First rib
32 Second rib
33 Posterior scalene muscle
34 Lung (left)
35 Esophagus

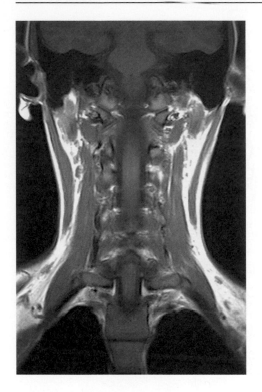

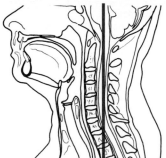

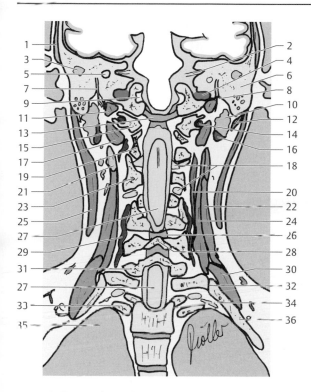

1 Temporal muscle
2 Internal acoustic meatus
3 Mastoid antrum
4 Jugular foramen
5 Vestibule
6 Mastoid process
7 Facial nerve canal
8 Stylomastoid foramen
9 Hypoglossal canal
10 Parotid gland
11 Rectus capitis lateralis muscle
12 Splenius capitis muscle
13 Transverse ligament
14 Vertebral artery
15 Atlas (posterior arch)
16 Digastric muscle (posterior belly)
17 Obliquus capitis inferior muscle
18 Spinal nerve roots
19 Inferior articular process (C2)
20 Spinalis cervicis muscle
21 Longissimus capitis muscle
22 Anterior scalene muscle
23 Superior articular process (C3)
24 Levator scapulae muscle
25 Sternocleidomastoid muscle
26 Ligamentum flavum
27 Spinal cord
28 Arch of C6 vertebra
29 Vertebral artery
30 Scalenus medius muscle
31 Transverse process (C7)
32 Costotransverse joint (T1)
33 Second rib (head)
34 Thoracic nerve (T1)
35 Lung (right)
36 First rib

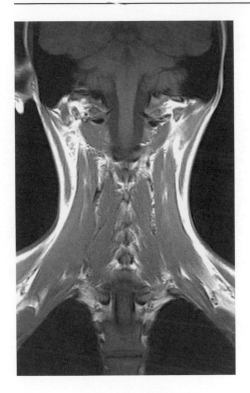

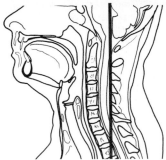

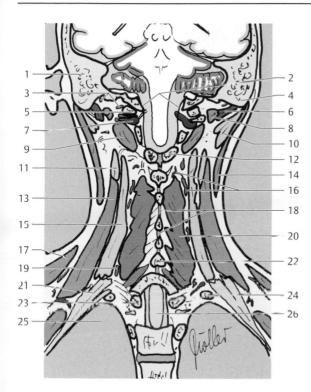

 1 Mastoid process (petrous part
    of temporal bone)
 2 Foramen magnum
 3 Suboccipital venous plexus
 4 Mastoid process
 5 Atlas (posterior arch)
 6 Digastric muscle (posterior
    belly)
 7 Vertebral artery
 8 Obliquus capitis superior
    muscle
 9 Obliquus capitis inferior
    muscle
10 Splenius capitis muscle
11 Longissimus capitis muscle
12 Spinous process (C2)
13 Levator scapulae muscle
14 Sternocleidomastoid muscle
15 Splenius cervicis muscle
16 Deep cervical artery and vein
17 Trapezius muscle
18 Interspinous ligaments
19 Deep cervical vein
20 Multifidus muscle
21 Brachial plexus
22 Spinous process (C7)
23 Costal process
24 First rib
25 Lung (right)
26 Spinal cord

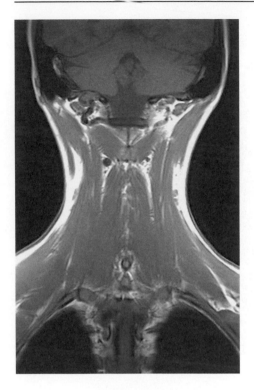

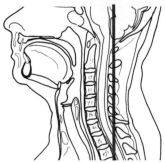

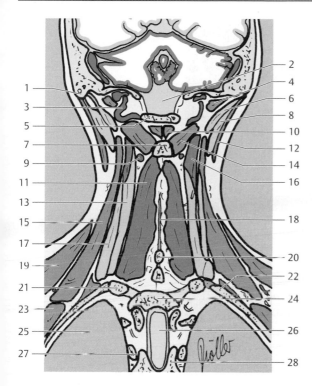

1 Mastoid process
2 Cisterna magna
3 Deep cervical vein
4 Obliquus capitis superior muscle
5 Atlas (posterior arch)
6 Longissimus capitis muscle
7 Spinous process of axis (C2)
8 Splenius capitis muscle
9 Deep cervical vein
10 Rectus capitis posterior major muscle
11 Semispinalis cervicis muscle
12 Sternocleidomastoid muscle
13 Longissimus cervicis muscle
14 Obliquus capitis inferior muscle
15 Levator scapulae muscle
16 Semispinalis capitis muscle
17 Splenius cervicis muscle
18 Supraspinous and interspinous ligaments
19 Trapezius muscle
20 Spinous process (C7)
21 Transverse process (T2)
22 Second rib
23 Supraspinatus muscle
24 Vertebra (T2)
25 Lung (right)
26 Spinal cord
27 Transverse process (T4)
28 Vertebra (T4)

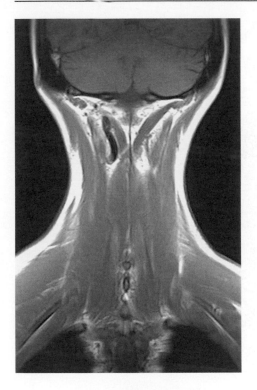

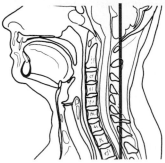

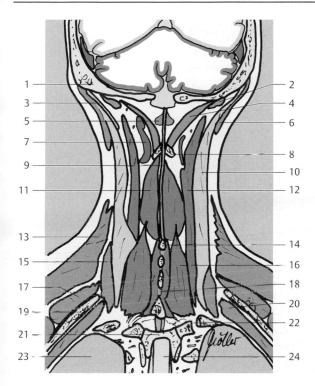

1 Occipital bone
2 Obliquus capitis superior muscle
3 Longissimus capitis muscle
4 Rectus capitis posterior major muscle
5 Rectus capitis posterior minor muscle
6 Sternocleidomastoid muscle
7 Deep cervical vein
8 Spinous process of axis (C2)
9 Nuchal ligament
10 Splenius capitis muscle
11 Semispinalis cervicis muscle
12 Semispinalis capitis muscle
13 Trapezius muscle
14 Spinous process
15 Rhomboid muscle
16 Multifidus muscle
17 Levator scapulae muscle
18 Interspinous ligament
19 Second rib
20 Intercostal muscle
21 Arch of T3 vertebra
22 Costotransverse joint (T3)
23 Lung (right)
24 Spinal cord

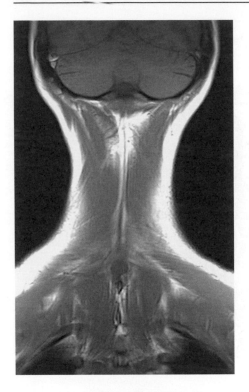

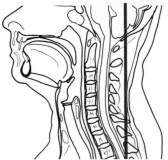

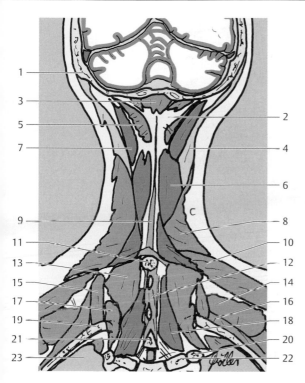

1 Occipital bone
2 Suboccipital fatty tissue
3 Rectus capitis posterior minor muscle
4 Splenius capitis muscle
5 Rectus capitis posterior major muscle
6 Semispinalis cervicis muscle
7 Semispinalis capitis muscle
8 Trapezius muscle, descending part (superior part)
9 Nuchal ligament
10 Trapezius muscle, transverse part (middle part)
11 Spinous process (C7)
12 Interspinous ligament
13 Splenius cervicis muscle
14 Levator scapulae muscle
15 Rhomboid muscle
16 Intercostal muscle
17 Serratus posterior superior muscle
18 Multifidus muscle
19 Third rib
20 Costotransverse joint (T4)
21 Spinous process (T3)
22 Costal process (T4)
23 Lung (right)

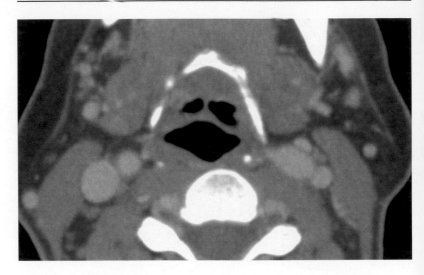

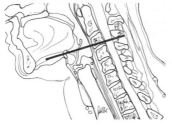

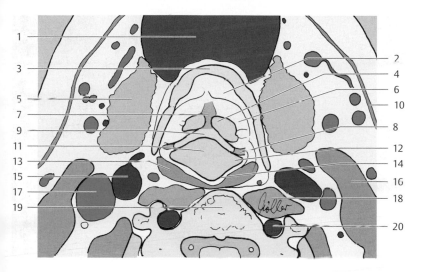

1 Muscles of tongue base
2 Pre-epiglottic space
3 Hyoid bone
4 Vallecula of epiglottis
5 Submandibular gland
6 Paraglottic space (visceral space)
7 Median glosso-epiglottic fold
8 Lateral glosso-epiglottic fold
9 Epiglottis (free edge)
10 Platysma

11 Hypopharynx
12 Piriform sinus
13 Middle pharyngeal constrictor muscle
14 Posterior wall of pharynx
15 Common carotid artery
16 Sternocleidomastoid muscle
17 Internal jugular vein
18 Longus colli muscle
19 C 3 cervical vertebra
20 Vertebral artery

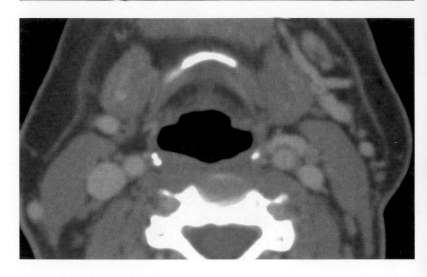

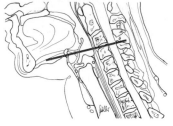

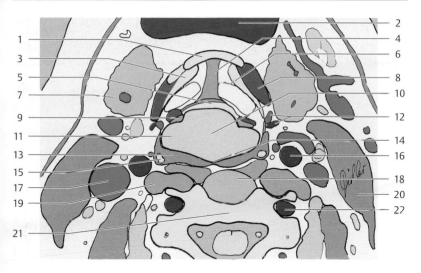

1 Hyoid bone
2 Muscles of tongue base
3 Pre-epiglottic space
4 Median glosso-epiglottic fold
5 Epiglottis
6 Paraglottic space
7 Submandibular gland
8 Sternohyoid and thyrohyoid
   muscles
9 Ary-epiglottic fold (with
   ary-epiglottic muscle)
10 Hypopharynx
11 Piriform sinus
12 Superior laryngeal artery and vein
13 Pharyngeal constrictor muscle
14 Thyrohyoid membrane
15 Superior horn of thyroid cartilage
16 Common carotid artery
17 Internal jugular vein
18 C3/C4 intervertebral disc
19 Longus colli muscle
20 Sternocleidomastoid muscle
21 C4 vertebral body
22 Vertebral artery

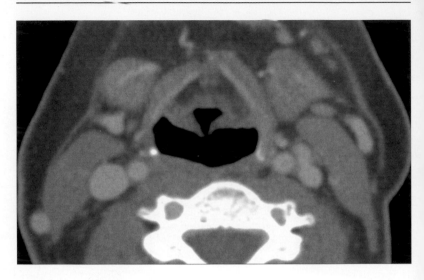

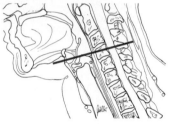

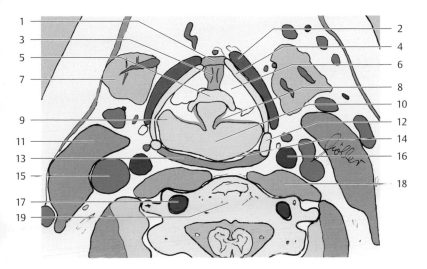

1 Median thyrohyoid ligament in superior thyroid notch
2 Infrahyoid muscles (sternothyroid, sternohyoid, thyrohyoid, omohyoid muscles)
3 Thyro-epiglottic ligament
4 Thyroid cartilage
5 Epiglottis, fixed part
6 Paraglottic space (visceral space)
7 Submandibular gland
8 Ary-epiglottic fold
9 Piriform sinus
10 Cavity of larynx
11 Sternocleidomastoid muscle
12 Superior horn of thyroid cartilage
13 Inferior pharyngeal constrictor muscle
14 Posterior wall of pharynx
15 Internal jugular vein
16 Common carotid artery
17 Vertebral artery
18 Longus colli muscle
19 C 4 vertebral body

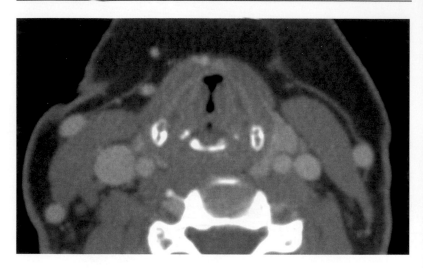

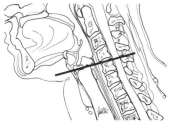

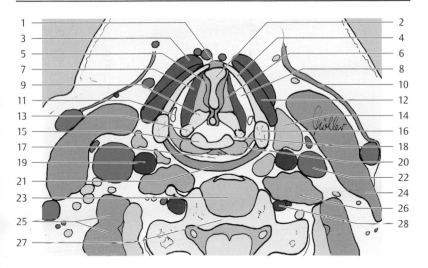

1 Laryngeal prominence
2 Glottis
3 Sternohyoid muscle
4 Thyroid cartilage
5 Vocal ligament ("true vocal cord")
6 Vocalis muscle
7 Thyro-arytenoid muscle
8 Paraglottic space (visceral space)
9 Arytenoid cartilage (vocal process)
10 Platysma
11 Piriform sinus (apex)
12 Thyrohyoid muscle
13 Arytenoid cartilage (muscular process)

14 Thyroid gland
15 Cricoid cartilage
16 Inferior horn of thyroid cartilage
17 Hypopharynx
18 Joint between cricoid cartilage and arytenoid cartilage
19 Common carotid artery
20 Posterior crico-arytenoid muscle
21 Inferior pharyngeal constrictor muscle
22 Internal jugular vein
23 C4/C5 intervertebral disc
24 Sternocleidomastoid muscle
25 Middle and posterior scalene muscles
26 Longus colli muscle
27 C5 cervical vertebra
28 Vertebral artery

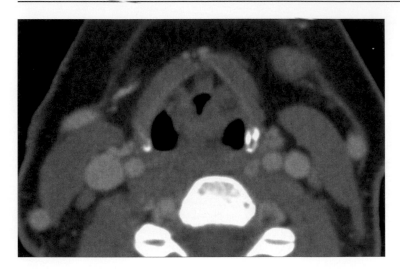

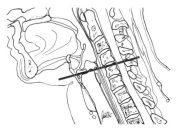

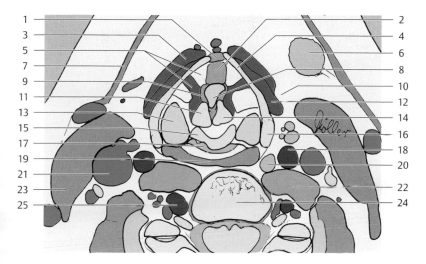

1   Median thyrohyoid ligament in
    superior thyroid notch
2   Pre-epiglottic space
3   Sternohyoid muscle
4   Thyroid cartilage
5   Paraglottic space (visceral
    space)
6   Submandibular gland
7   Platysma
8   Laryngeal inlet
9   Vestibular fold ("false vocal
    cord")
10 Anterior cervical space
11 Vocal process of arytenoid
    cartilage
12 Thyrohyoid muscle

13 Piriform sinus
14 Arytenoid cartilage
15 Cricoid cartilage
16 Posterior (partially calcified) border
    of thyroid cartilage
17 Posterior crico-arytenoid muscle
18 Common carotid artery
19 Inferior pharyngeal constrictor
    muscle
20 Thyroid gland
21 Internal jugular vein
22 Longus colli muscle
23 Sternocleidomastoid muscle
24 C 4 cervical vertebra
25 Vertebral artery

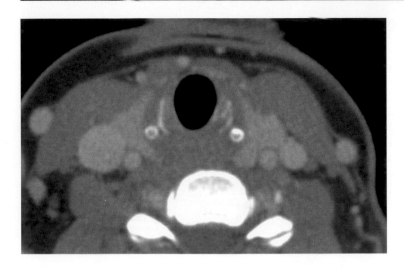

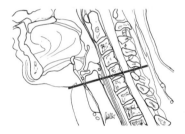

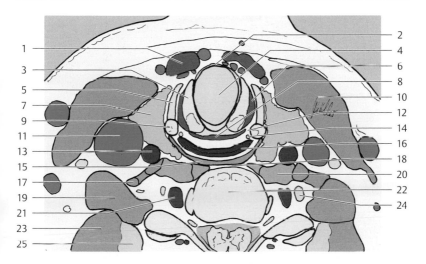

1 Sternohyoid muscle
2 Cricothyroid ligament (median)
3 Cricoid cartilage
4 Laryngeal cavity
5 Thyroid cartilage
6 Cricothyroid muscle
7 Thyroid gland
8 Posterior crico-arytenoid muscle
9 Inferior horn of thyroid cartilage
10 Sternocleidomastoid muscle
11 Internal jugular vein
12 Cricothyroid space
13 Common carotid artery
14 Recurrent laryngeal nerve
15 Inferior pharyngeal constrictor muscle
16 Hypopharynx (laryngopharynx), junction with esophagus
17 Anterior scalene muscle
18 Retropharyngeal space
19 Middle scalene muscle
20 Longus colli muscle
21 Vertebral artery
22 C5 vertebra
23 Posterior scalene muscle
24 C5 spinal nerve
25 Longissimus capitis muscle

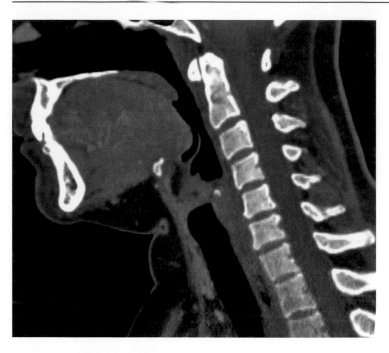

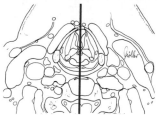

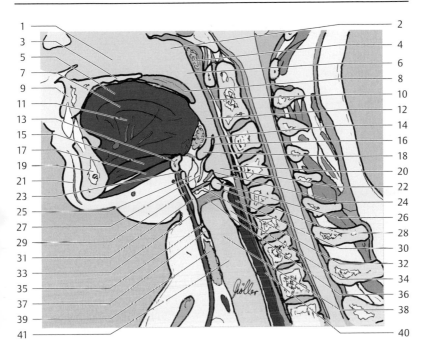

1   Nasal cavity
2   Pharyngeal cavity (fornix)
3   Hard palate
4   Pharyngeal tonsil
5   Superior longitudinal muscle of tongue
6   Nasopharynx
7   Inferior longitudinal muscle of tongue
8   Soft palate
9   Maxilla
10 Longus colli muscle
11 Genioglossus muscle
12 Oropharynx (oral cavity)
13 Hyoid bone
14 Lingual tonsil
15 Geniohyoid muscle
16 Epiglottis (free edge)
17 Mylohyoid muscle
18 Vallecula of epiglottis
19 Mandible
20 Hypopharynx (posterior wall)
21 Platysma
22 Laryngopharynx (hypopharynx)
23 Thyrohyoid ligament
24 Ary-epiglottic fold
25 Pre-epiglottic fat pad
26 Arytenoid cartilage
27 Epiglottis (fixed part)
28 Crico-arytenoid joint
29 Thyrohyoid muscle
30 Inferior pharyngeal constrictor muscle
31 Thyroid cartilage
32 Vestibular fold ("false vocal cord")
33 Sternohyoid muscle
34 Cricoid cartilage (lamina)
35 Cricothyroid ligament
36 Vocal fold (vocal cord)
37 Cricoid cartilage (arch)
38 Larynx (subglottic space)
39 Thyroid gland
40 Esophagus
41 Trachea

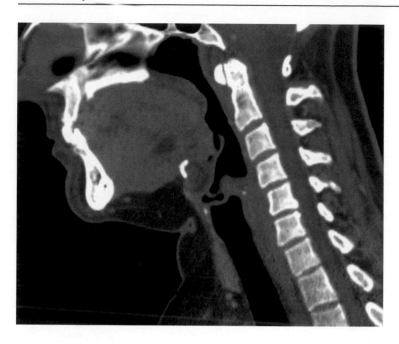

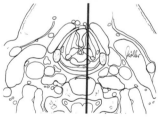

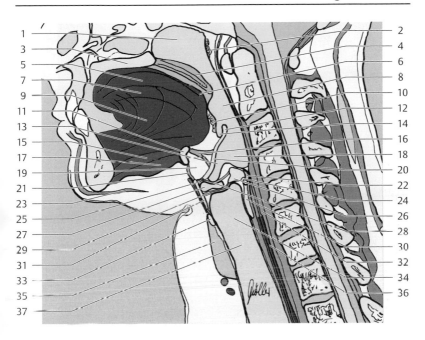

1   Nasopharynx
2   Pharyngeal tonsil
3   Hard palate
4   Soft palate
5   Superior longitudinal muscle of tongue
6   Lingual aponeurosis
7   Inferior longitudinal muscle of tongue
8   Oropharynx (oral cavity), mesopharynx
9   Genioglossus muscle
10 Lingual tonsil
11 Hyoid bone
12 Epiglottis (free edge)
13 Laryngeal vestibule
14 Epiglottic vallecula
15 Geniohyoid muscle
16 Hyo-epiglottic ligament
17 Mylohyoid muscle
18 Hypopharynx (laryngopharynx)
19 Pre-epiglottic fat pad
20 Epiglottis (fixed part)
21 Median thyrohyoid ligament
22 Transverse and oblique arytenoid muscle
23 Platysma
24 Crico-arytenoid joint
25 Thyro-epiglottic ligament
26 Arytenoid cartilage
27 Laryngeal ventricle
28 Vestibular fold ("false vocal cord")
29 Vocal fold (vocal cord)
30 Cricoid cartilage (lamina)
31 Thyroid cartilage
32 Inferior pharyngeal constrictor muscle
33 Cricoid cartilage (arch)
34 Larynx (subglottic space)
35 Thyroid gland
36 Esophagus
37 Trachea

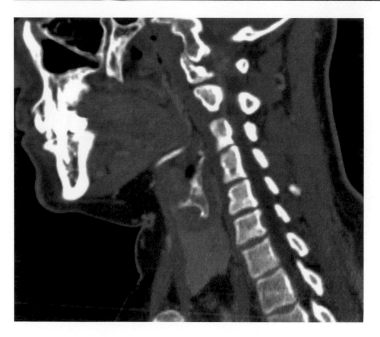

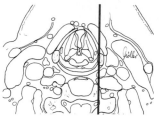

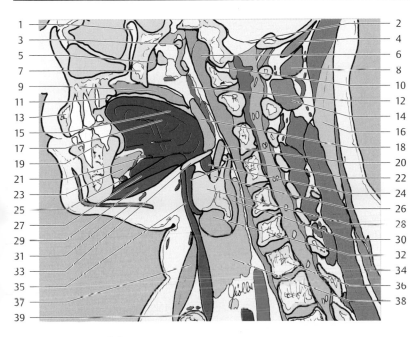

1 Greater palatine groove
2 Foramen magnum
3 Pharyngeal recess
4 Rectus capitis posterior minor muscle
5 Tensor veli palatini muscle
6 Longus capitis muscle
7 Pterygoid process (medial plate, hamulus)
8 Rectus capitis posterior major muscle
9 Soft palate
10 Atlanto-occipital joint
11 Oral cavity
12 Pharyngeal plexus (pharyngeal venous plexus)
13 Maxilla
14 Obliquus capitis inferior muscle
15 Longitudinal superior muscle of tongue
16 Splenius capitis muscle
17 Inferior longitudinal muscle of tongue
18 Hyoglossus muscle
19 Mandible
20 Middle pharyngeal constrictor muscle
21 Lingual artery
22 Thyroid cartilage (superior horn)
23 Sublingual gland
24 Thyrohyoid muscle
25 Deep lingual artery and vein
26 Piriform recess
27 Mylohyoid muscle
28 Thyroid cartilage
29 Digastric muscle (anterior belly)
30 Inferior pharyngeal constrictor muscle
31 Platysma
32 Cricothyroid muscle
33 Hyoid bone
34 Trapezius muscle
35 Sternohyoid muscle
36 C 6 cervical vertebra
37 Sternocleidomastoid muscle
38 Thyroid gland
39 Sternum

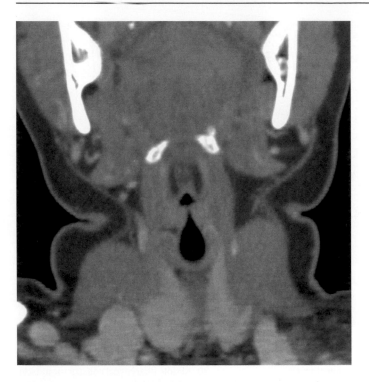

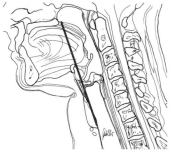

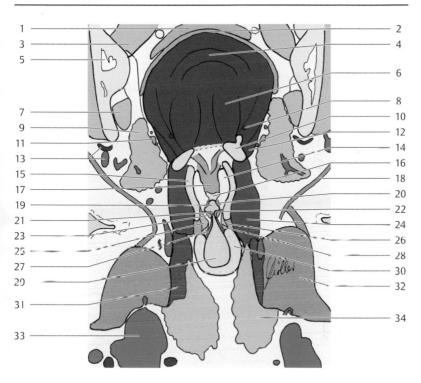

1 Soft palate
2 Oropharynx (oral cavity)
3 Lateral pterygoid muscle
4 Transverse lingual muscle
5 Mandible
6 Genioglossus muscle
7 Medial pterygoid muscle
8 Lingual artery
9 Submandibular gland
10 Hyoid bone
11 Digastric muscle (tendon)
12 Hyoglossus muscle
13 Facial artery and vein
14 Pre-epiglottic fat pad
15 Thyroid cartilage
16 Epiglottis
17 Median thyrohyoid ligament

18 Platysma
19 Laryngeal ventricle
20 Vestibular fold ("false vocal cord")
21 Rima glottidis (glottic aperture)
22 Vocal fold (vocal cord)
23 Vocalis muscle
24 Thyrohyoid muscle
25 Thyro-arytenoid muscle
26 Cricothyroid ligament
27 Conus elasticus
28 Crico-arytenoid muscle
29 Larynx (subglottic space)
30 Cricoid cartilage
31 Sternohyoid muscle
32 Sternocleidomastoid muscle
33 Internal jugular vein
34 Thyroid gland

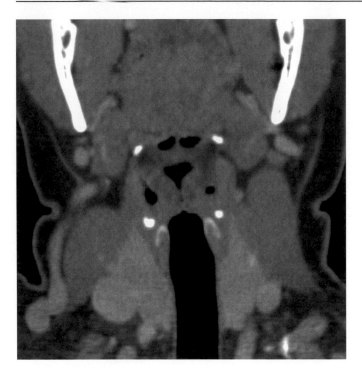

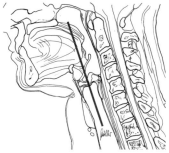

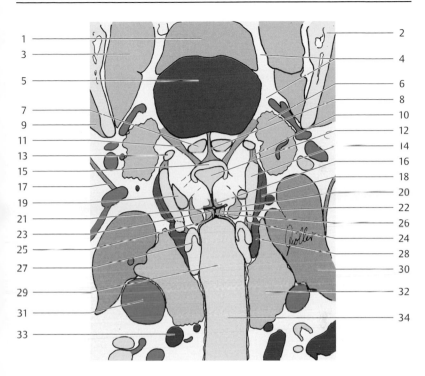

1 Soft palate
2 Mandible
3 Medial pterygoid muscle
4 Parapharyngeal space
5 Tongue
6 Submandibular gland
7 Epiglottic vallecula
8 Median glosso-epiglottic fold
9 Masseter muscle
10 Lateral thyrohyoid ligament
11 Lateral glosso-epiglottic fold
12 Larynx (supraglottic space)
13 Hyoid bone
14 Thyroid cartilage
15 Epiglottis
16 Vestibular fold ("false vocal cord")
17 Platysma

18 Thyrohyoid muscle
19 Piriform sinus
20 Thyro-arytenoid muscle
21 Laryngeal ventricle
22 Vocalis muscle
23 Vocal fold (vocal cord)
24 Cricothyroid ligament
25 Conus elasticus
26 Rima glottidis (glottic aperture)
27 Cricoid cartilage
28 Cricothyroid muscle
29 Larynx (subglottic space)
30 Sternocleidomastoid muscle
31 Internal jugular vein
32 Thyroid gland
33 Common carotid artery
34 Trachea

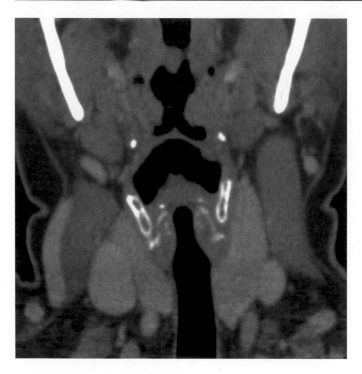

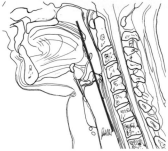

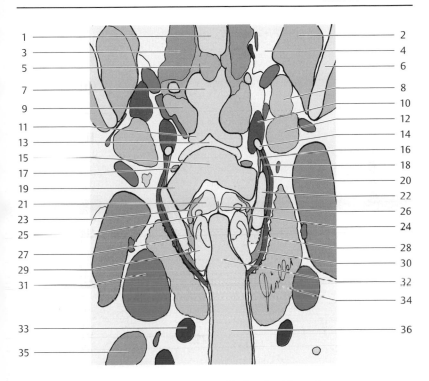

1 Nasopharynx
2 Medial pterygoid muscle
3 Palatopharyngeus muscle
4 Parapharyngeal space
5 Soft palate with uvula
6 Mandible
7 Oropharynx
8 Styloglossus muscle
9 Palatine tonsil
10 Digastric muscle
11 Epiglottic vallecula
12 Submandibular gland
13 Epiglottis
14 Hyoid bone
15 Larynx (supraglottic)
16 Thyrohyoid membrane
17 Ary-epiglottic fold
18 Thyrohyoid muscle
19 Piriform sinus

20 Omohyoid muscle
21 Arytenoid cartilage
22 Thyroid cartilage
23 Thyro-arytenoid muscle
24 Crico-arytenoid muscle (lateral)
25 Crico-arytenoid joint
26 Intercartilaginous fold
27 Cricothyroid muscle
28 Sternothyroid muscle
29 Cricoid cartilage
30 Inferior pharyngeal constrictor
    muscle
31 Internal jugular vein
32 Larynx (subglottic)
33 Common carotid artery
34 Thyroid gland
35 Anterior scalene muscle
36 Trachea

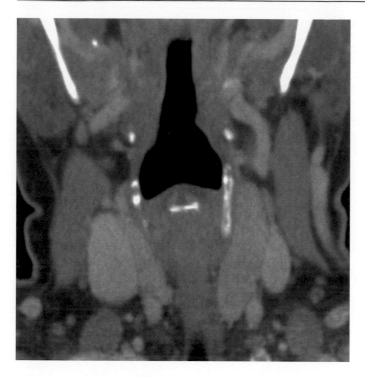

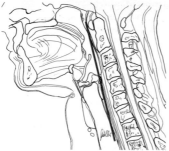

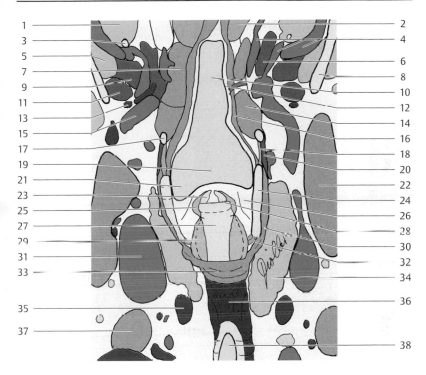

1 Parotid gland
2 Longus colli muscle
3 Styloid process
4 Pharyngeal venous plexus
5 Medial pterygoid muscle
6 Stylohyoid muscle
7 Palatopharyngeus muscle
8 Maxillary nerve (V₂)
9 Styloglossus muscle
10 Oropharynx
11 Digastric muscle
12 Mucosa of pharynx
13 Facial artery
14 Stylopharyngeus muscle
15 Facial vein
16 Middle pharyngeal constrictor muscle
17 Hyoid bone
18 Thyrohyoid membrane
19 Hypopharynx
20 Thyrohyoid muscle
21 Piriform sinus (apex)
22 Sternocleidomastoid muscle
23 Arytenoid cartilage (muscular process)
24 Thyroid cartilage
25 Thyro-arytenoid muscle
26 Cricothyroid space
27 Cricoid cartilage (lamina)
28 Crico-arytenoid joint
29 Crico-arytenoid muscle (posterior)
30 Inferior pharyngeal constrictor muscle, thyropharyngeal part
31 Internal jugular vein
32 Cricothyroid joint
33 Inferior pharyngeal constrictor muscle, cricopharyngeal part
34 Thyroid gland
35 Common carotid artery
36 Esophagus
37 Anterior scalene muscle
38 Trachea

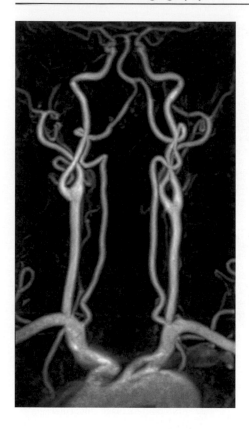

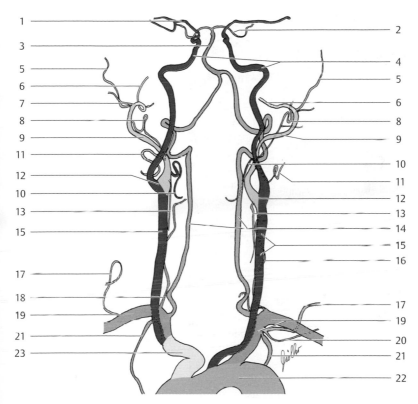

1 Middle cerebral artery
2 Posterior cerebral artery
3 Basilar artery
4 Internal carotid artery
5 Superficial temporal artery
6 Maxillary artery
7 Posterior auricular artery
8 Occipital artery
9 External carotid artery
10 Lingual artery
11 Facial artery
12 Carotid bifurcation
13 Superior thyroid artery
14 Vertebral artery
15 Common carotid artery
16 Inferior thyroid artery
17 Ascending cervical artery
18 Thyrocervical trunk
19 Subclavian artery
20 Supreme intercostal artery
21 Internal thoracic artery
22 Aortic arch
23 Brachiocephalic trunk

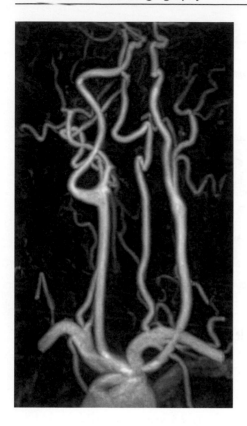

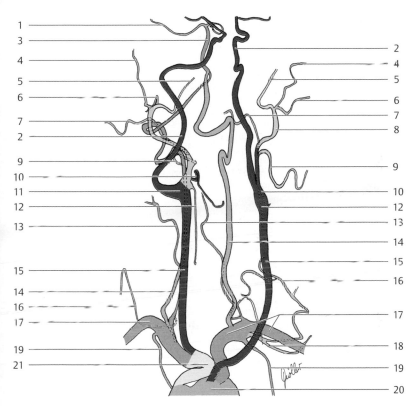

1 Posterior cerebral artery
2 Internal carotid artery
3 Basilar artery
4 Superficial temporal artery
5 Maxillary artery
6 Posterior auricular artery
7 Occipital artery
8 External carotid artery
9 Facial artery
10 Lingual artery
11 Carotid bifurcation
12 Superior thyroid artery
13 Inferior thyroid artery
14 Vertebral artery
15 Common carotid artery
16 Ascending cervical artery
17 Subclavian artery
18 Supreme intercostal artery
19 Internal thoracic artery
20 Aortic arch
21 Brachiocephalic trunk

Bibliography

Basset LW, Gold RU, Seeger LL. MRI Atlas of the Musculoskeletal System. Köln:-Deutscher Ärzte-Verlag;1989

Beyer-Enke SA, Tiedemann K, Görich J, et al. Dünnschichtcomputertomographie der Schädelbasis. Radiologe 1987;27:438–488

Braun H, Kenn W, Schneider S, et al. Direkte MR-Arthrographie des Handgelenkes. Röfo 2003;175:1515–1524

Bulling A, Castrop F, Agneskirchner J, et al. Body Explorer 2.0. Heidelberg: Springer Electronic Media; 2001

Burgener FA, Aeyers SP, Tan RK. Differential Diagnosis in MRI. Stuttgart: Thieme; 2002

Cahill DR, Orland MJ, Reading CC. Atlas of Human Cross-Sectional Anatomy. New York:Wiley-Liss;1995

Chacko AK, Katzberg RW, MacKay A. MRI Atlas of Normal Anatomy. New York: McGraw-Hill; 1991

Clavero JA, Alomar X, Monill JM, et al. MR imaging of ligament and tendon injuries of the fingers. Radiographics 2002;22:237–256

Clavero JA, Golano P, Farinas O, Alomar X, Monill JM, Espligas M. Extensor mechanism of the fingers: MR imaging—anatomic correlation. Radiographics 2003;23:593–611

Connell DA, Koulouris G, Thorn DA, Potter HG.Contrast-enhanced MR angiography of the hand. Radiographics 2002; 22:583–599

Dauber W. Pocket Atlas of Human Anatomy. 5th ed. Stuttgart: Thieme; 2007

Delfaut EM, et al. Imaging of foot and ankle entrapment syndromes. Radiographics 2003; 23:613–623

El-Khoury GY, Bergman RA, Montgomery EJ. Sectional Anatomy by MRI/CT. New York: Churchill-Livingstone; 1990

El-Khoury GY. Essentials in Musculoskeletal Imaging. New York:Churchill Livingstone; 2003

Fishbein NJ, Dillon WP, Barkovich AJ. Teaching Atlas of Brain Imaging. Stuttgart: Thieme; 2000

Garcia-Valtuille R, Abascal F, Cerezal L, et al. Anatomy and MR imaging appearances of synovial plicae of the knee. Radiographics 2002; 22:775–784

Grumme T, Kluge W, Kretzmar K, Roesler A. Zerebrale und spinale CT. Berlin: Blackwell;1998

Han, M-C, Kim C-W. Sectional Human Anatomy. Ilchokak: Seoul, Korea; 1989

Harnsberger R. Diagnostic Imaging. Head and Neck. Salt Lake City, Utah: Amirsys; 2006

Harnsberger R, Osborne A, Macdonald A, Ross J. Imaging Anatomy. Salt Lake City, Utah: Amirsys; 2006

Hosten N, Liebig T. CT of the Head and Spine. Stuttgart: Thieme; 2002

Huk WJ, Gademann G, Friedmann G. MRI of Central Nervous System Diseases. Berlin: Springer; 1990

Kahle W, Frotscher M. Color Atlas and Textbook of Human Anatomy. Vol. 3: Nervous System and Sensory Organs. 6th ed. Stuttgart: Thieme; 2010

Kang MS, Resnick D. MRI of the Extremities: An Anatomic Atlas. Philadelphia:-Saunders; 2002

Koritke JG, Sick H. Atlas of Sectional Human Anatomy. Urban & Schwarzenberg, Baltimore 1988

Kretschmann H-J, Weinrich W. Cranial Neuroimaging and Clinical Neuroanatomy. Stuttgart: Thieme; 2003

Leblanc A. Encephalo-peripheral Nervous System. Berlin: Springer; 2001

Leonhardt H, Tillmann B. Töndury G, Zilles K, eds. Bewegungsapparat. (Rauber/ Kopsch Anatomie des Menschen. Lehrbuch und Atlas. Vol. I.) Stuttgart: Thieme; 1987

Lustrin ES, Karakas SP, Ortiz AO, et al. Pediatric cervical spine: Normal anatomy, variants, and trauma. Radiographics 2003; 23:539–560

Mayerhöfer ME, Breitenseher MJ. MR-Diagnostik der lateralen Sprunggelenksbänder. Röfo 2003; 175:670–675

Mengiardi B, Zanetti M, Schottle PB, et al. Spring ligament complex: MR imaging–anatomic correlation and findings in asymptomatic subjects. Radiology 2005; 237:242–249

Meschan I. Synopsis of Radiologic Anatomy. Philadelphia: Saunders; 1978

Mohana-Borges AV, Theumann NH, Pfirrmann CWA, Chung CB, Resnick DL, Trudell DJ. Lesser metatarsophalangeal joints. Radiology 2003; 227:175–182

Moeller TB, Reif F. MR Atlas of the Musculoskeletal System. Boston: Blackwell Science; 1994

Moeller TB, Reif E, Neuroradiologische Schnittbilddiagnostik. Constance: Schnetztor; 2002

Moeller TB, Reif E. Pocket Atlas of Radiographic Anatomy. Stuttgart: Thieme; 2000

Morag Y, Jacobson JA, Shields G, et al. MR Arthrography of rotator interval, long head of the biceps brachii, and biceps pulley of the shoulder. Radiology 2005; 235:21–30

Munshi, M, Pretterklieber ML, Chung CB, et al. Anterior bundle of ulnar collateral ligament: evaluation of anatomic relationship by using MR imaging, MR arthrography, and gross anatomic and histologic analysis. Radiology 2004; 231:797–803

Netter FH. Atlas of Human Anatomy. 5th ed. Philadelphia: Saunders; 2011

Nowicki BH, Haughton VM. Neural foraminal ligament of the lumbar spine: appearance at CT and MR imaging. Radiology 1992; 183:257–264

Oae K, Takao M, Naito K, et al. Injury of the tibiofibular syndesmosis: value of MR imaging for diagnosis. Radiology 2003; 227:155–161

Pech P, Daniels DL, Williams AL, Haughton VM. The cervical neural foramina: correlation of microtomy and CT anatomy. Radiology 1985; 155:143–146

Platzer W. Color Atlas and Textbook of Human Anatomy. Vol.1: Locomotor System. 6th ed. Stuttgart: Thieme; 2008

Rauber A, Kopsch F. Anatomie des Menschen. Vol. III: Nervensystem, Sinnesorgane. Stuttgart. Thieme; 1987

Richter E, Feyerabend T. Normal Lymph Node Topography. Berlin: Springer; 1991

Robinson P, White LM. Soft-tissue and osseous impingement syndromes of the ankle. Radiographics 2002; 22:1457–1471

Runmeny EJ, Reimer P, Heindel W. MR Imaging of the Body. Stuttgart: Thieme; 2008

Sartor K: Neuroradiologie. 2nd ed. Stuttgart: Thieme; 2001

Schäfer FKW, et al. [Sport injuries of the extensor mechanism of the knee]. Radiologe 2002; 42:799–810

Schmitt R, Lanz U. Diagnostic Imaging of the Hand. Stuttgart: Thieme; 2007

Schnitzlein HN, Reed Murtagh F. Imaging Atlas of the Head and Spine. Baltimore: Urban & Schwarzenberg; 1990

Schünke M, Schulte E, Schumacher U, Ross LM, Lamperti ED. THIEME Atlas of Anatomy Series. Stuttgart: Thieme; 2010

Schuenke M, Schulte E, Ross LM, Lamberti ED. Thieme Atlas of Anatomy. General Anatomy and Musculoskeletal System. Stuttgart: Thieme; 2006

Stark DD, Bradley WG. Magnetic Resonance Imaging. St. Louis: Mosby; 1999

Strobel K, Hodler J. MRT des Kniegelenkes. Radiologie up2date. Stuttgart: Thieme; 2003

Stoller DW. MRI, Arthroscopy, and Surgical Anatomy of the Joints. Philadelphia: Lippincott Williams & Wilkins; 1999

Stoller DW, Tirman B. Diagnostic Imaging: Orthopaedics. Salt Lake City, Utah: Amirsys; 2004

Theumann NH, et al. MR Imaging of the metacarpophalangeal joints of the fingers. Radiology 2002; 222:437–445

Theumann NH, et al. Extrinsic carpal ligaments: Normal MR arthrographic appearance in cadavers. Radiology 2003; 226:171–179

Tiedemann K. Anatomy of the Head and Neck. Weinheim: VCH;1993

Uhlenbrock D. MR Imaging of the Spine and Spinal Cord. Stuttgart: Thieme; 2004

Vahlensieck M, Linneborn G, Schild HH, Schmidt HM. MRT der Bursae des Kniegelenk. Röfo 2001; 173:195–199

Vahlensieck M. Anatomie der Schulterregion. Radiologe 2004; 44:556–561

Vahlensieck M, Reiser M. MRT des Bewegungsapparates. Stuttgart: Thieme; 2001

Von Hagens G, Romreil LJ, Ross MH, Tiedemann K. The Visible Human Body. Philadelphia: Lea & Febinger; 1991

Wegener OH. Ganzkörper-Computertomographie. 2nd ed. Blackwell: Berlin; 1992

Index